ASTHMA
CURRENT PERSPECTIVES

G. Mac Cochrane BSc, MB, BS, FRCP
Consultant Physician and Honorary Senior Lecturer
Guy's Hospital
London, England

William F. Jackson MA, MB, BChir, MRCP
Medical Writer
Formerly Honorary Consultant
Department of Medicine
Guy's Hospital
London, England

P. John Rees MA, MD, MB, BChir, FRCP
Consultant Physician and Senior Lecturer in Medicine
United Medical and Dental Schools of Guy's and St. Thomas's Hospitals
London, England

with contributions on childhood asthma from

John O Warner MD FRCP DCH
Professor of Child Health
University of Southampton/Southampton General Hospital
Southampton, England

Presented as a service to medicine by

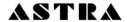

Astra Draco AB, PO Box 34, S-221 00 Lund, Sweden

ACKNOWLEDGEMENTS

We gratefully acknowledge the help of a number of colleagues and organisations who allowed us to borrow illustrations to fill the gaps in our own collections or provided the inspiration for artwork:

Crown Copyright, **1.9, 1.10, 1.11, 1.12** (Crown Copyright is reproduced with the permission of the Controller of HMSO); G. Jelke, Schleswig, Germany, **2.2**; A. Laitinen and L. A Laitinen, Helsinki, Finland, **2.3, 3.10, 16.3, 16.4**; P.K. Jeffery, London, England, **2.4, 2.7, 2.8, 2.9**; E. Ädelroth, Umeå, Sweden, **2.7, 2.8**; P.J Barnes, London, England, **3.1, 3.2, 3.6, 3.11, 3.13, 3.14**; Clinical Vision Ltd, Harwell, England, **3.1, 3.2, 3.6, 3.11, 3.13, 3.14, 16.22**; Veisland, The Medical Image Bank, Malmö, Sweden, **3.4, 3.5, 3.8, 3.9**; J. Erjefält, Lund, Sweden, **3.12**; H. Stammberger, Graz, Austria, **5.7**; G. D'Amato, Naples, Italy, **6.7**; S. Durham, London, England, **6.13**; C. Mims, London, England, **6.14**; J. Sanderson, London, England, **6.16**; W. Owen, London, England, **6.17**; T. Lee, London, England, **7.3, 7.4**; F.E. Hargreave, Hamilton, Canada, **7.5**; C. O'Callaghan, Leicester, England, **10.4, 10.12, 10.15**; E. Berg, Lund, Sweden, **10.9**; Racal Ltd, **11.1**; P. Le Souëf, Perth, Australia, **15.8, 16.24**; R. K. Gregson, Southampton, England, **15.11**; Group for Asthma Management and Education, Southampton Schools, **15.14**; D.L Marsh, Harwell, England, **16.19**.

ISBN 0 7234 2454 3

Cataloguing in Publication Data

CIP catalogue records are available from the British library and the Library of Congress.

Acquisitions Editor:	Claire Hooper
Project Manager:	Moira Sarsfield
Design:	Marie McNestry
Layout:	Marie McNestry
	Lee Riches
	Chris Read
Illustration:	Richard Prime

Originated by Reed Reprographics
Produced by The KPC Group, London and Ashford, Kent.
Printed and bound in the United Kingdom

CONTENTS

PREFACE

Evidence from around the world shows that the prevalence of asthma is increasing, and in many countries it is the commonest significant chronic condition of childhood. Pathological studies have shown the importance of inflammation of the airway wall in asthma of all grades of severity, and inflammatory changes have been shown to persist even when symptoms are quiescent. The recognition of the persistence of the asthmatic tendency into adult life suggests that the rising prevalence of asthma in childhood will lead to an acceleration of the increasing adult problem.

The current perspectives covered in this book range from the basic scientific aspects of asthma to the practical clinical areas of everyday management. Exciting information is emerging on the cellular interactions in the airway wall and the role of a wide range of mediators in the inflammation and symptomatology of asthma. This new understanding is already influencing the practicalities of management, and we have tried to reflect this in what, for many busy clinicians, may be the most immediately important part of the book – the sections on management.

We have reviewed the groups of drugs commonly used in asthma management, and the various drug delivery systems, and we have summarised some of the recent work on the performance characteristics of different inhalers. We have discussed guidelines for the management of acute and chronic asthma in adults and children. This is an ever changing area, where consensus statements on management struggle to keep pace with the development of new drugs and new devices to deliver them. We have also considered practical clinical problems outside the standard stepwise approaches to management, including complementary therapy, patient education and compliance, and the management of asthma in special situations and particular groups of patients.

We have included a wide range of graphs, art work, colour photographs, radiographs and tables, with the aim of producing an approachable, easily readable book which will help in the delivery of appropriate care in asthma, and which will have worldwide applications. We hope that the book will be of practical value to all those concerned with the care of patients with asthma.

Most of the illustrations in the book come from our own collections, but others have been generously loaned to us by friends and colleagues. They are acknowledged in detail elsewhere, and we thank them all for their help. We particularly thank John Warner for his major contribution to the sections on childhood asthma, and the staff of Mosby-Wolfe – especially Moira Sarsfield – for the speedy and efficient manner in which the book has been progressed to publication.

GMC, WFJ, PJR

1 EPIDEMIOLOGY OF ASTHMA

DEFINITION

Asthma is most simply defined as:

A disorder characterised by narrowing of airways which is reversible with time, either spontaneously or as a result of treatment.

A more detailed definition is that proposed in the International Consensus Report on the Diagnosis and Management of Asthma (*Clin Exper Allergy* 1992; **22 (Suppl 1)**: S1–S72):

Asthma is a chronic inflammatory disorder of the airways in which many cells play a role, in particular mast cells and eosinophils. In susceptible individuals, this inflammation causes symptoms that are usually associated with widespread but variable airflow obstruction that is often reversible either spontaneously or with treatment and causes an associated increase in airway responsiveness to a variety of stimuli.

Although airway responsiveness is not usually routinely investigated in clinical practice, this more detailed definition has now been widely adopted. It is valuable in focusing on both the inflammatory nature and the potential reversibility of asthma, and thus in suggesting the most appropriate forms of therapy. It is, however, not an all-embracing definition, as asthma can still be characterised in a number of different ways (**Fig. 1.1**). At present, it is not possible to characterise asthma by biochemical or genetic features, but there is much continuing research in these fields.

Airway hyperresponsiveness (AHR) was identified as a feature of asthma in the 1960s, and challenge tests with substances which provoke bronchoconstriction, such as histamine and methacholine, have been an important research tool in the investigation of mechanisms in asthma, and of responses to therapy, over the past 25 years (*see* Chapter 4). In a clinical setting, AHR is suggested by a history of immediate symptoms on exposure to smoke, cold air, exercise or dust.

In the past, many believed that AHR was the fundamental mechanism in asthma but, as the inflammatory nature of asthma became clear in the 1980s, further research suggested that AHR is usually a consequence of airway inflammation rather than a primary process.

It has also become clear that many environmental, and most genetic influences in asthma, probably act mainly by provoking airway inflammation, rather than by direct stimulation of AHR (**Fig. 1.2**).

Despite general agreement about the relationship between airway inflammation, AHR and reversible airflow

Characteristic features of asthma	
Clinical	Wheeze and/or cough Nocturnal symptoms
Physiological	Reversibility of airways' obstruction Airway hyperresponsiveness (AHR)
Immunological (in some patients)	Positive skinprick tests Elevated serum IgE level
Pathological	Sputum eosinophilia (in some patients) Desquamative eosinophilic airway inflammation (on biopsy)
Biochemical	None
Genetic	None

Fig. 1.1. Characteristic features of asthma.

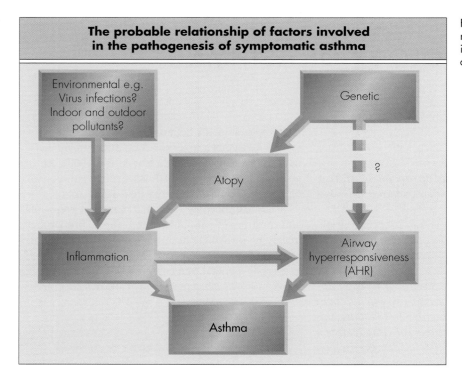

The probable relationship of factors involved in the pathogenesis of symptomatic asthma

Fig. 1.2. The probable relationship of factors involved in the pathogenesis of symptomatic asthma.

Environmental e.g. Virus infections? Indoor and outdoor pollutants?

Genetic

Atopy

?

Inflammation

Airway hyperresponsiveness (AHR)

Asthma

Some problems in the definition of asthma

- Recurrent but infrequent wheezing occurs at some stage in up to 40% of children. Is this always asthma?

- Is 'wheezy bronchitis' in children asthma?

- Is recurrent nocturnal coughing in childhood in the absence of known infection always indicative of asthma?

- Is reversible airflow obstruction always diagnostic of asthma?

- What are the boundaries between chronic obstructive pulmonary disease (COPD) and asthma in adult patients?

- Which investigations should be used to assess the severity and reversibility of airflow obstruction?

- Does the presence of airway hyperresponsiveness (AHR) always imply asthma?

- Can asthma be present without airway hyperresponsiveness?

- In severe chronic asthma, reversibility of airflow obstruction may be slight or absent

Fig. 1.3. Some problems in the definition of asthma.

obstruction in asthma, a number of factors complicate the definition of asthma (**Fig. 1.3**). In particular, chronic uncontrolled asthma is associated with structural changes in the airway wall, which lead to a progressive reduction in the scope for reversibility of airflow obstruction. Thus, patients with severe chronic asthma may show little or no reversibility of airflow obstruction.

The differential diagnosis of asthma is further discussed in Chapters 8 and 14.

TYPES OF ASTHMA

Asthma is often classified as *extrinsic*, in which identifiable external trigger factors are present, or *intrinsic*, in which no such factors are identified. Typically, most children with asthma have identifiable trigger factors, whereas most patients with asthma which begins in adult life do not, and this has obvious relevance in the management of patients.

Current understanding of the role of genetic factors, inducers and triggers in asthma has made it obvious that this classification is an over-simplification. It is more clinically useful to consider a number of different variants of asthma (**Fig. 1.4**).

ASTHMA SEVERITY

There is no universally agreed classification of the severity of asthma, but a commonly used grading is shown in **Fig. 1.5**.

Most patients have mild or very mild asthma, and the medical, social and financial costs of asthma are inversely related to its severity. Studies in several countries have shown that the total direct and indirect financial costs attributable to the 20% of patients with very severe and

Types of asthma	
Type	Common features
Childhood onset	Patient usually atopic, marked variability, obvious trigger factors
Adult onset	Demonstrable atopy uncommon, usually persistent, infection a common trigger, but other identifiable triggers uncommon
Occupational	Under-diagnosed, careful assessment needed
Nocturnal	May occur in all other types of asthma, indicates poor overall control and increased AHR
Prominent cough	A common presentation in childhood, may precede significant airflow obstruction, responsive to anti-inflammatory treatment
Exercise-induced	A common precipitant of other types of asthma, especially in childhood May be the main problem in childhood

Fig. 1.4. Types of asthma.

Severity of asthma: classification and frequency		
Severity	Features	% of total asthma population
Very severe	• Disabling disease • Numerous exacerbations with hospital admission • Much time off work or school • Life-threatening attacks	2
Severe	• Daily wheezing • Severe nocturnal symptoms • Poor quality of life • Off work or school for several weeks per year • Hospital admission common	18
Moderate	• Daily symptoms, but no significant diurnal variation • Occasional nocturnal symptoms • Patient avoids exercise	20
Mild	• Periodic symptoms • Patient reacts to triggers (e.g. pollen or cold air) • Symptoms restrict activity 2–3 times per week	20
Very mild	• Occasional cough or wheezing that does not cause major impairment • Respiratory tract sensitive to infections and intense cold • Allergens may cause symptoms	40

Fig. 1.5. Severity of asthma: classification and frequency.

severe asthma may be as much as 60% of the total national expenditure on asthma (**Fig. 1.6**). Most of these costs result from emergency care and in-patient treatment in hospital.

The costs associated with the appropriate preventive management of patients with mild and moderate asthma are relatively low. The cost of mortality is not included in the figures shown in **Fig. 1.6** and, as most asthma deaths occur in patients with severe disease,

these figures understate the true cost to society of very severe and severe asthma.

EPIDEMIOLOGY

The impact of asthma on health and quality of life is substantial, especially in the developed world. It has been estimated that the total prevalence of asthma is

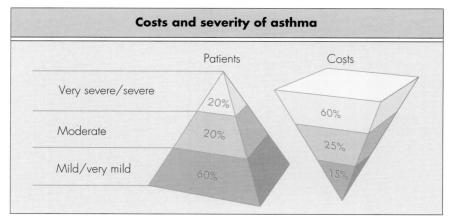

Costs and severity of asthma

Fig. 1.6. The costs resulting from asthma are inversely related to its severity. The most severely affected 20% of patients may account for up to 60% of the total national expenditure on asthma, while the least severely affected 60% may account for only 15%.

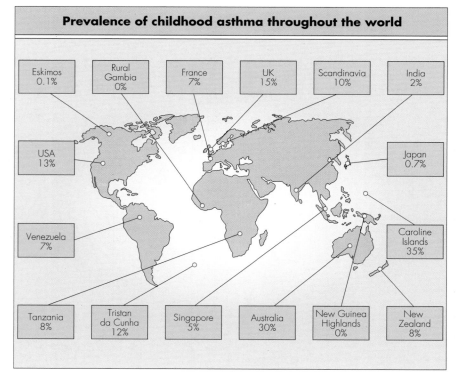

Prevalence of childhood asthma throughout the world

Fig. 1.7. The prevalence of childhood asthma throughout the world. The figures cited here are best estimates, but in some countries, such as the UK and Australia, different studies have shown widely differing results. These differences relate in part to the difficulty of classification of asthma in childhood; some studies probably include more children with 'wheezy bronchitis' than others. It is clear, however, that there are real differences in the prevalence of childhood asthma between different countries. Prevalence may be affected by genetic factors (as in Tristan da Cunha), by climatic conditions, by degree of urbanisation and by other currently unknown factors.

Prevalence of asthma: changes over time

Country	Age group (years)	Years studied	Wheeze prevalence	Asthma prevalence	Reference
Australia	8–10	1982 and 1992	13→24%	7→11%	Peat *et al., Br Med J* 1994;**308**: 1591–6
Scotland	8–13	1964 and 1989	10→20%	4→10%	Ninan and Russell, *Br Med J* 1992; **304**: 873–5
Wales	12	1973 and 1988	17→22%	4→9%	Burr *et al., Arch Dis Child.* 1989;**64**: 1452–6
Australia	Adult	1981 and 1990	18→29%	9→16%	Peat *et al., Br Med J.* 1992 **305**: 1326–9

Fig. 1.8. Prevalence of asthma: changes over time.

around 7.2% of the world population (about 100 million individuals), with a world population prevalence of about 6% in adults and 10% in children. At least 40,000 deaths per year worldwide can probably be attributed to asthma.

The estimated prevalence of asthma varies in different regions of the world (**Fig. 1.7**), and in different parts of each country. In general, asthma is more common in urban than in rural areas.

The prevalence of asthma in children and adults has been shown to be increasing in several recent studies (**Fig. 1.8**). The number of reported new cases of asthma has usually been greatest in younger patients. These increases are supported by studies in England which show increased self-reporting of asthma, an increase in the number of episodes of asthma requiring a general medical consultation (**Fig. 1.9**) and a progressive increase in the number of prescriptions for asthma therapy (**Fig. 1.10**). Broadly similar increases have been found in studies in other developed countries. For example, the Australian childhood study summarised in **Fig. 1.8** showed that the percentage of all children who used some form of medication for asthma rose from 7% to 25% between 1982 and 1992.

A greater awareness of asthma, and of the possibility of successful treatment, has undoubtedly resulted in some 'diagnostic transfer' from other respiratory conditions to asthma, but this is unlikely to be the sole explanation for the increase in reported prevalence, as the prevalence of wheezing (**Fig. 1.8**) and of shortness of breath have also increased. No study has reported a decline in asthma prevalence.

There has been a progressive increase in hospital admissions from asthma in all age groups, and particularly in infancy, throughout the developed world. Whilst some of the increase may be explained by greater accuracy in diagnosis, and by a shift in the balance of care,

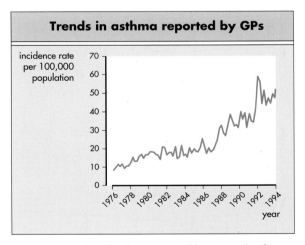

Fig. 1.9. Episodes of asthma reported by a sample of general medical practices in the weekly returns service of the Royal College of General Practitioners. The mean weekly incidence is plotted in 12-week periods. The base is the entire population of England and Wales. The sharp rises seen in 1987 and 1991 may be partly artefactual (due to the inclusion of new practices at these times), but the overall rising trend in the incidence rate of asthma episodes is clear.

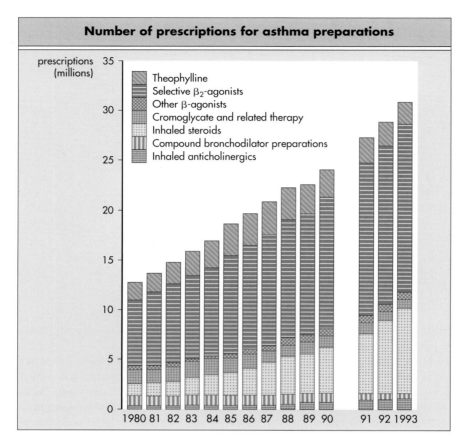

Number of prescriptions for asthma preparations

prescriptions (millions)

Legend:
- Theophylline
- Selective β_2-agonists
- Other β-agonists
- Cromoglycate and related therapy
- Inhaled steroids
- Compound bronchodilator preparations
- Inhaled anticholinergics

Years: 1980 81 82 83 84 85 86 87 88 89 90 91 92 1993

Fig. 1.10. Number of prescriptions for asthma preparations in England from 1980–1993. Data from 1980–1990 are based on dispensing fees, while those from 1991–1993 are based on items dispensed. Some of these medications may have been dispensed for other pulmonary disease, especially COPD. In 1993, inhaled steroids accounted for more than 25% and selective β_2-agonists for more than 50% of all asthma preparation prescriptions, so that together they were over 80% of the total. Prescriptions for both groups have increased rapidly; for inhaled steroids by more than six times over the period covered. (Source: Prescription Pricing Authority, analysis by Department of Health, England and Wales.)

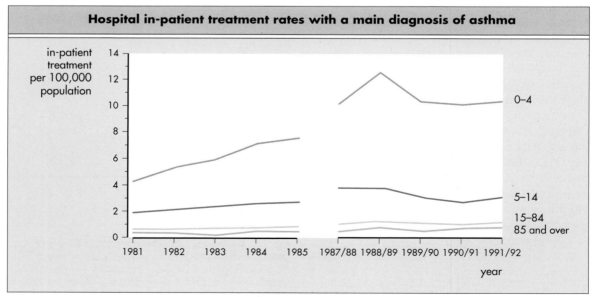

Hospital in-patient treatment rates with a main diagnosis of asthma

in-patient treatment per 100,000 population

Age groups: 0–4, 5–14, 15–84, 85 and over

Years: 1981 1982 1983 1984 1985 1987/88 1988/89 1989/90 1990/91 1991/92

year

Fig. 1.11. Hospital in-patient treatment rates with a main diagnosis of asthma in England. The basis of data collection changed in 1986, but the trend to an increased admission rate, especially in children, during the 1980s is clear. The admission rate during the early 1990s shows signs of a plateau. This could reflect a decline in acute episodes, or the more successful treatment of acute episodes outside hospital. (Source: Department of Health.)

with increasing reliance on hospital rather than primary medical care, there may also be other factors involved. In England, at least, this increase seems to have levelled out during the 1990s (**Fig. 1.11**).

The most alarming feature of the increased prevalence of asthma has been an apparent trend during the 1980s towards an increased mortality rate from the disease (**Fig. 1.12**). This trend has been noted worldwide. Most 'asthma' deaths in developed countries occur in older people (**Fig. 1.13**). The increase in asthma mortality largely reflects the growth in the number of elderly people in the population, but audit studies have shown that asthma deaths in patients of all ages often reflect sub-optimal care.

Two peaks in asthma mortality in New Zealand over the past 30 years caused particular concern, and have been the subject of particularly detailed investigation. The cause of these epidemics is still unresolved, although there are strong suggestions of a relationship between death and the over-use of inhaled β-agonist drugs, or the inappropriate use of these drugs without accompanying anti-inflammatory therapy. Progressive airway inflammation may be masked where long-term symptomatic treatment with β_2-agonists is prescribed without accompanying anti-inflammatory therapy.

There are suggestions from some studies that a greater use of anti-inflammatory prophylactic compounds, with a consequent lesser dependence on β_2-agonists as core therapy for asthma, may be associated with a fall in the mortality rate from the disease. The greater use of inhaled anti-inflammatory therapy in England (**Fig. 1.10**) may have contributed to the encouraging 20% fall in the number of deaths from asthma in patients below the age of 65 in England which occurred between 1984–6 and 1990–2 (**Fig. 1.12**).

GENETICS AND ENVIRONMENT IN ASTHMA

The increased prevalence of asthma is probably the result of a combination of genetic and environmental factors.

Asthma is highly correlated with atopy (**Fig. 1.14** and page 18), and there has been a recent unexplained increase in the prevalence of atopy in many populations. Some recent studies suggest that bronchial hyper-responsiveness and a major locus controlling IgE production are both located in one or more genes on Chromosome 5q31–q33. Even in the presence of an inherited predisposition, many other factors also affect the development of atopy and its effects in the individual patient (**Fig. 1.15**). Genetic effects on the fetal immune response may be influenced by maternal smoking, nutrition and disease, so allergic mothers are more likely to have allergic babies than allergic fathers.

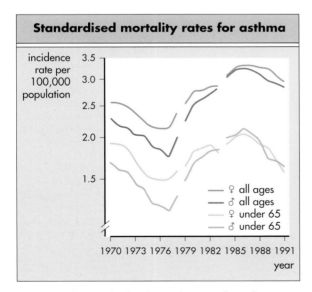

Fig. 1.12. The standardised mortality rates for asthma in England from 1970 to 1991. The rates are calculated using a 3-year average plotted against the middle year of the average. Discontinuities in the graphs mark points at which the basis of data collection and analysis changed. (Source: Office of Population Censuses and Surveys.)

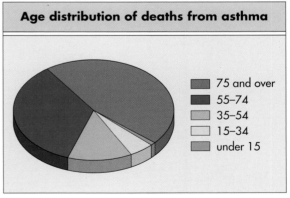

Fig. 1.13. The age distribution of deaths from asthma in England in 1991. The high proportion of deaths in the age groups 55–74 and 75 and over may, in part, reflect inappropriate diagnostic labelling, but fatal asthma in the young is now very uncommon. (Source: Office of Population Censuses and Surveys.)

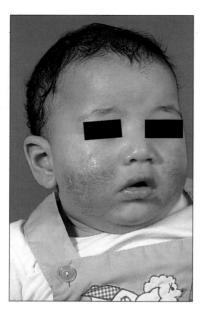

Fig. 1.14. Infantile atopic eczema. This 7-month-old boy shows the facial involvement which is common at this age, with large areas of eczema on the cheeks, but sparing of the peri-oral region. Asthma is highly correlated with atopy, especially in children.

Other environmental factors may have an influence on the development or expression of atopy as asthma. These include increased exposure to allergens – especially house dust mite antigens (*see* page 33) – and to occupational sensitisers. It is possible that respiratory infections in early childhood may induce asthma, but there are also suggestions that early exposure to some childhood infections may protect against atopy and asthma.

Increased exposure to tobacco smoke in infancy may also be relevant, but there is more debate about the role of outdoor pollutants. Atmospheric pollutants can trigger exacerbations in patients with established asthma, but there is no evidence that atmospheric pollution can induce asthma in a previously non-susceptible patient. For example, a comparison between highly-polluted Leipzig and less-polluted Munich showed a significantly higher prevalence of asthma in Munich.

Inducers and triggers of asthma are further discussed in Chapter 6.

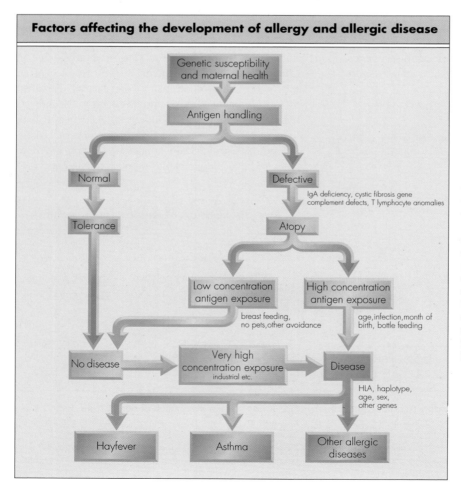

Factors affecting the development of allergy and allergic disease

Fig. 1.15. The inter-relationship between factors which affect the development of allergy and allergic disease. Genetic susceptibility and maternal health influences the handling of antigen by the fetus and its immune response. If this is defective, allergy can develop, leading to the atopic state. Disease may not develop if subsequent antigen exposure is low in concentration and occurs at an appropriate time. However, high levels of exposure, with the adjuvant effects of infection and pollution, lead to the development of allergic disease, the nature of which is influenced by other genes, age and sex. Very high antigen exposure might lead to disease even in non-atopic individuals.

2 PATHOLOGY OF ASTHMA

Originally, most information on the pathology of asthma was derived from post-mortem studies of patients who had died from asthma, and thus had severe disease; however some information was also available from post-mortem studies on patients with known asthma who died from another cause.

More recently, biopsy samples have been obtained in studies of patients with asthma of various grades of severity. Rigid bronchoscopy allows the removal of larger biopsy samples than fibreoptic bronchoscopy (**Fig. 2.1**), but the fibreoptic bronchoscope can penetrate further into the bronchi than the rigid bronchoscope, and fibreoptic bronchoscopy is less traumatic for the patient, so this technique is most commonly used. Other lung biopsy methods are of little value in asthma.

At a macroscopic level, bronchoscopy often confirms the inflammatory nature of asthma (**Fig. 2.2**), and microscopic studies on biopsy samples have confirmed that inflammatory changes can be seen in asthma of all grades of severity, including recently diagnosed asthma (**Fig. 2.3**). The quantitative assessment of cells and mediators in biopsy and bronchoalveolar lavage (BAL) samples confirms the early involvement of inflammation in asthma of all degrees of severity (*see* Chapter 3).

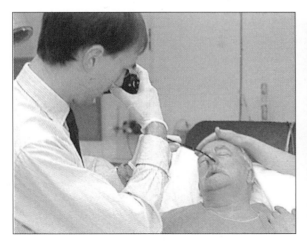

Fig. 2.1. Fibreoptic bronchoscopy. Bronchoscopy is not a routine procedure in patients with asthma, but it can be used in formal investigations to obtain small bronchial biopsies or to obtain bronchoalveolar lavage fluid (BAL) for investigation of its cell and mediator content. Special precautions must be taken to prevent the induction of bronchoconstriction by bronchoscopy. These include atropine premedication, prior use of a nebulised β_2-agonist, adequate local anaesthesia to the pharynx and careful monitoring during and after the procedure.

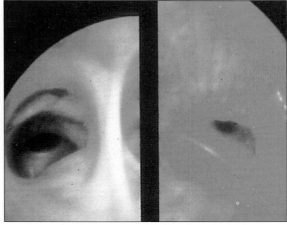

Fig. 2.2. The inflammatory nature of asthma can often be seen on bronchoscopy, as in this comparison of a normal patient (left) and a patient with asthma (right). Even 'mild' asthma is commonly associated with the inflammatory changes seen on the right: the asthmatic mucosa is reddened and oedematous.

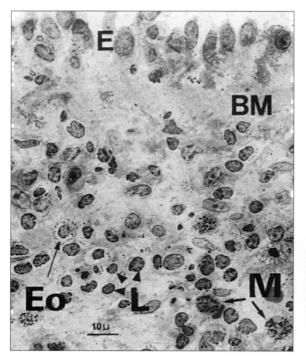

Fig. 2.3. The inflammatory nature of asthma can be confirmed on electron microscopy. This section of the airway wall comes from a patient with asthma of 9 months' duration, who had received only symptomatic treatment with a β_2-agonist. The airway epithelium (E) is severely damaged, and an intense inflammatory reaction can be seen beneath the basement membrane (BM). Several types of inflammatory cells can be identified, including eosinophils (Eo), lymphocytes (L) and degranulated mast cells (M).

In the early stages, the inflammatory processes in asthma are potentially reversible, as no permanent structural change has occurred (*see* **Figs 16.3, 16.4**).

Other abnormalities which may be found at relatively early stages in asthma include oedema of the airway wall, shedding of the airway epithelium (**Figs 2.4, 2.5, 2.9, 2.11**) and mucus plugging of the airway lumen (**Fig. 2.5**). Although these processes may be associated with severe symptoms, they are also potentially reversible with effective anti-inflammatory treatment.

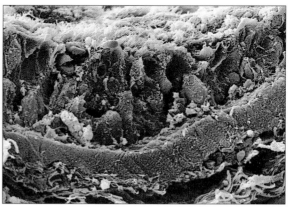

Fig. 2.4. Scanning electron microscopic (SEM) image of the damaged surface epithelium, and the consistently thickened reticular layer of the basement membrane, in the bronchus of a subject with a history of chronic asthma, who died of a non-respiratory cause (original magnification x2000).

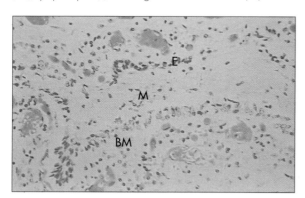

Fig. 2.5. Mucus plugging and epithelial shedding are commonly found in asthma of all grades of severity. This section of a small airway (original magnification x40) shows a mucus plug (M), disruption and denudation of the epithelial layer (E), thickening of the reticular basement membrane (BM) and some inflammatory cell infiltration of the airway wall. Compare these appearances with those of a normal small airway (**Fig. 2.6**). Changes of this severity are potentially reversible with effective treatment.

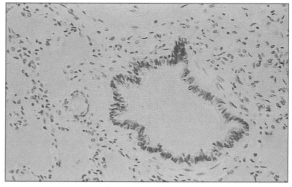

Fig. 2.6. Normal small airway. In contrast to **Fig. 2.5**, this section shows an empty airway, with a well-defined epithelium. The airway epithelium is surrounded by a normal basement membrane and a normal smooth muscle layer, and there is no inflammatory cell infiltrate.

Chronic asthma is associated with other structural changes which are less easily reversed. A relatively early finding is thickening of the reticular layer of the basement membrane (**Figs 2.4, 2.6, 2.7, 2.8, 16.5**) and this is accompanied by goblet cell hyperplasia (**Figs 2.7, 2.8**), new vessel formation and vasodilatation in the smooth muscle layer, hyperplasia and hypertrophy of the airway smooth muscle (**Fig. 2.9**), mucous gland hypertrophy, and ultimately the development of irreversible fibrosis.

Occasionally, extensive mucus plugs are coughed up by patients, with immediate lessening of obstructive symptoms (**Fig. 2.10**).

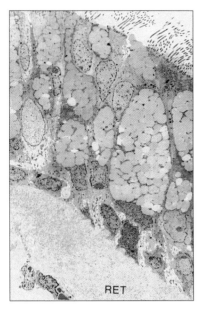

Fig. 2.7. Thickened reticular basement membrane (RET) and goblet cell hyperplasia in the airway wall of a patient with mild asthma. This electron micrograph was prepared from a biopsy obtained by fibreoptic bronchoscopy (original magnification x1950). Compare these appearances with those of a normal small airway (Fig. 2.8).

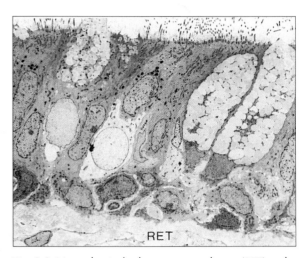

Fig. 2.8. Normal reticular basement membrane (RET) and epithelium in a healthy control subject. Compare the appearance with that of the small airway of a patient with mild asthma (Fig. 2.7).

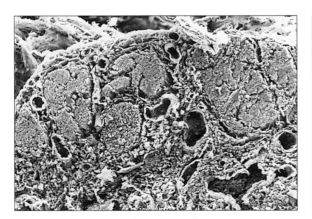

Fig. 2.9. Scanning electron microscopic (SEM) image of the thickened airway wall in a patient who died from asthma. The surface epithelium has been lost completely and the wall is grossly thickened by enlargement of the bronchial smooth muscle mass (arrows) and bronchial vasodilatation (original magnification x350).

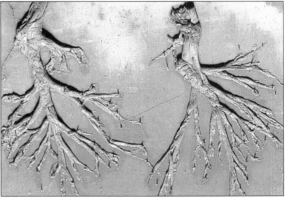

Fig. 2.10. Mucus plugs from patients with asthma. Sometimes patients with asthma cough up firm, rubbery mucus plugs which can be teased out into casts of the airways, as in these examples. The expectoration of such large plugs may be associated with considerable relief of symptoms. Similar plugs are commonly found at post-mortem in patients dying of severe asthma.

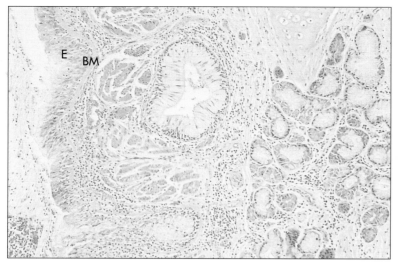

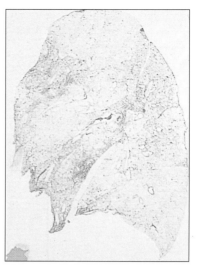

Fig. 2.11. Large airway wall from a fatal case of asthma (original magnification x25). The lumen is to the left, and it contains a mucus plug. The epithelium (E) is disrupted, the basement membrane (BM) is thickened, there is widespread infiltration with inflammatory cells, smooth muscle hyperplasia and hypertrophy of the mucus glands (to the right).

Fig. 2.12. Whole lung slice in a fatal case of asthma. There is generalised hyperinflation, but no significant destruction of the alveolar walls.

At post-mortem in patients who die from asthma, the medium-sized and small airways are usually occluded by tenacious plugs of exudate and secretions, containing eosinophils and epithelial cells, which are firmly attached to the damaged bronchial epithelial surface. Histologically, the bronchial wall shows areas of denudation of epithelium, areas of epithelial regeneration, generalised gross oedema and severe submucosal inflammation with an infiltrate in which eosinophils are abundant (**Fig. 2.11**).

Macroscopically, the lungs from fatal cases of asthma usually show sustained hyperinflation but, in contrast to the appearance in emphysema, there is no destruction of the alveolar walls (**Fig. 2.12**).

The pathological changes in the airways in asthma are summarised in **Fig. 2.13**.

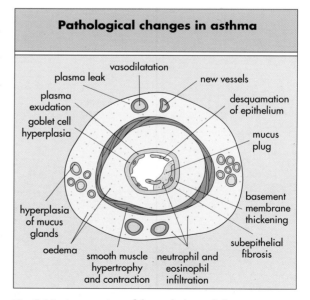

Pathological changes in asthma

Fig. 2.13. An overview of the pathological changes in asthma. All these changes contribute to airway narrowing. The increase of resistance is not linearly related to the size of the airway lumen; it is related to the fourth power of the radius of the lumen, so a comparatively small change in airway calibre can produce large changes in airflow.

3 MECHANISMS IN ASTHMA

Asthma is usually regarded as an allergic condition, and many patients develop symptoms in response to allergens such as house dust mites or pollen grains; but often, especially in adult patients, there are no obvious underlying allergies. It is now clear that many provoking factors are involved in the development of asthma symptoms, and these can be divided into two main groups: inducers and triggers.

- *Inducers* of asthma include genetic factors, allergies, infections and, probably, other factors related to occupational background or environmental influences. They act mainly by inducing airway inflammation, which leads to airway hyperresponsiveness (AHR) and asthma symptoms.
- *Triggers* of asthma are factors which cause airway smooth muscle contraction and asthma symptoms on a background of pre-existing airway inflammation and AHR. These include a wide range of stimuli such as exercise, cold air, irritants, smoke, pollutants, β-blocking drugs and stress and, in susceptible individuals, drugs such as aspirin and other non-steroidal anti-inflammatories, foods and other inhaled or ingested substances.

The clinical role of inducers and triggers in asthma is further discussed in Chapter 6.

At a cellular level, the mechanisms of asthma seem to be similar whatever its cause. There does not appear to be any fundamental difference between allergic and non-allergic asthma; both involve the same combination of inflammation and AHR, and both are potentially susceptible to the same pharmacological approaches.

The 'traditional' view of asthma, which was widely held until a few years ago, implicated the mast cell as the principal orchestrator of the asthmatic process. Inhaled allergen interacts with surface mast cells through IgE-dependent mechanisms, and this interaction leads to the release of mediators, such as histamine and leukotrienes, which then act on receptors on airway smooth muscle cells and lead to bronchoconstriction (**Fig. 3.1**).

Although a mechanism of this kind probably accounts for some of the immediate features of acute asthma, it is now clear that it cannot explain most of the recognised features of established, chronic asthma.

The current view of asthma regards it as a complex inflammatory condition involving many inflammatory cells, which release a wide variety of mediators. These mediators act on cells of the airway leading to smooth muscle contraction, mucus hypersecretion, plasma leakage, oedema, activation of cholinergic reflexes and activation of sensory nerves, which can lead to amplification of the ongoing inflammatory response (**Fig. 3.2**).

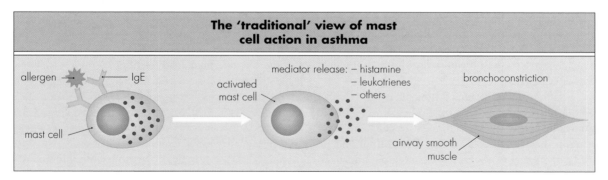

The 'traditional' view of mast cell action in asthma

allergen — IgE — activated mast cell — mediator release: – histamine – leukotrienes – others — bronchoconstriction — airway smooth muscle — mast cell

Fig. 3.1. The 'traditional' view of mast cell action in asthma. In the sensitised individual, mast cell surface-bound specific antibodies encounter allergen at its points of deposition in the body, such as the respiratory mucosa, and the resulting antigen–antibody binding (which is believed to involve the bridging of adjacent surface IgE molecules by divalent antigen) results in activation of the mast cell. The activated mast cell then releases mediators, including histamine and leukotrienes, into the surrounding tissue fluid, and these provoke bronchoconstriction by direct action on the airway smooth muscle. This is now recognised to be just one of many mechanisms in asthma; it does not account for the inflammatory features of the disorder.

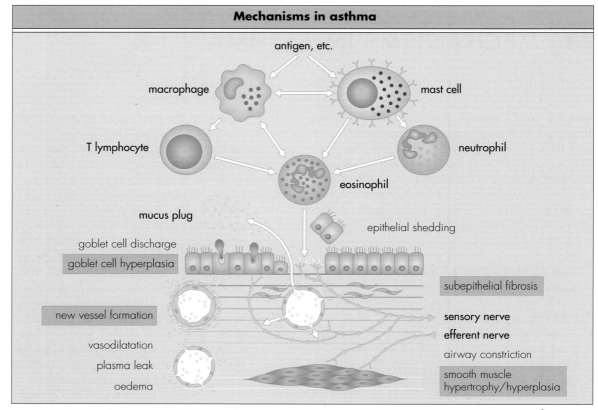

Mechanisms in asthma

Fig. 3.2. The current view of mechanisms in asthma.
Asthma is now viewed as a complex inflammatory condition involving many inflammatory cells, which release a wide variety of mediators. These mediators act on cells of the airway leading to potentially reversible abnormalities, including smooth muscle contraction, mucus hypersecretion, plasma leakage, oedema, activation of cholinergic reflexes and activation of sensory nerves, which can lead to amplification of the ongoing inflammatory response. Chronic inflammation also leads to structural changes (labelled in red in the figure), including goblet cell hyperplasia, new vessel formation, subepithelial fibrosis and smooth muscle hypertrophy and hyperplasia, which are less easy to reverse than the acute processes.

Chronic inflammation also leads to structural changes, such as goblet cell hyperplasia, subepithelial fibrosis and smooth muscle hypertrophy and hyperplasia (**Fig. 3.2**), which are less easy to reverse than the acute processes (*see* Chapter 2).

This new understanding of asthma has been reached on the basis of many *in vitro* studies, and of *in vivo* studies involving the measurement of cells and mediators in bronchoalveolar lavage (BAL) fluid and the study of biopsies by various microscopic and histochemical techniques.

SENSITISATION

A sensitisation process—which is likely to occur in early infancy—is believed to be the first stage in the development of asthma, as in other allergic disorders (**Fig. 1.15**).

Contact of an allergen with the respiratory mucosa for the first time may lead to sensitisation in a susceptible individual. This process involves the dendritic cells in the respiratory mucosa, together with T-helper (TH) lymphocytes and B lymphocytes (B cells) (**Fig. 3.3**). The dendritic cells act as antigen presenting cells, which sensitise a subset of T lymphocytes (T-helper cells). In an atopic host (an individual who has the predisposition for IgE immune responses), it is believed that sensitised T-helper 2 (TH2) cells signal B cells to produce IgE antibodies. The IgE produced by B cells is released into the circulation, and much of it becomes bound onto high affinity receptors on the surface of mast cells (which are abundant in the mucosa) and basophils (which circulate in the blood).

Sensitisation to inhaled allergen

allergen

dendritic cell

T cell

TH2 cell

TH1 cell

resting
B cells

IL-4
IL-13

IFN-γ

proliferation/
differentiation

activated B cell

IgE synthesis and release

Fig. 3.3. Sensitisation to inhaled allergen. The dendritic cells in the respiratory mucosa act as antigen presenting cells. In the regional lymph nodes, they sensitise subsets of T lymphocytes (T-helper cells). In an atopic host it is believed that the activation of IgE production and release is promoted by two cytokines, interleukin-4 (IL-4) and IL-13 (IL-13), which are released from TH2 cells. By contrast, type 1 T-helper lymphocytes (TH1 cells) release interferon-γ (IFN-γ), a cytokine which deactivates B cells and thus suppresses IgE release. The IgE produced by B cells is released into the circulation, and much of it becomes bound onto high affinity receptors on the surface of mast cells and basophils.

THE ROLE OF INDIVIDUAL CELL TYPES AND MEDIATORS

Mast cells

On subsequent allergen exposure in the sensitised individual, mast cell surface-bound specific antibodies encounter allergen at its points of deposition in the respiratory tract. The resulting antigen–antibody binding results in activation of the mast cell. The activated mast cell releases pre-formed mediators, especially histamine, and newly formed mediators, including leukotriene C_4 (LTC_4), prostaglandin D_2, bradykinin and platelet activating factor (PAF), into the surrounding tissue fluid (**Figs 3.4, 3.5**). These mediators are believed to be largely responsible for the airway constriction that results from contact with an allergen (**Fig. 3.1**). Mast cell activation is effectively blocked by β_2-agonist drugs but not by acute administration of steroids.

The mast cell is thus now believed to play an important role in the immediate response to allergen (and also to exercise and some other triggers of asthma), and in the early stages of airway inflammation, but it probably does not play a major role in the late response to allergen challenge (**Fig. 3.6**) or in chronic asthma.

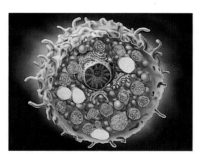

Fig. 3.4. Resting mast cell. This artist's representation of a cross section shows the typical appearance of the high number of secretory granules within the cell. On electron microscopy, these are electron dense. The granules contain different mediators and enzymes, including histamine, prostaglandins, leukotrienes, heparin, tryptase and chymase. 'Scrolls' in the particles are a sign of tryptase content. The organised structure of many of the granules is thought to be the result of strong ionic interactions between heparin, histamine and the cationic proteins tryptase and chymase. Arachidonic acid, the substrate for prostaglandin and leukotriene synthesis, is stored in distinct, featureless lipid bodies. The numerous folds extending from the cell surface are known as microplicae.

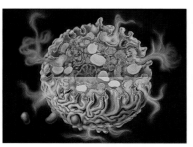

Fig. 3.5. Secreting mast cell. This artist's representation of a wedge section through the cell shows the effects of IgE–antigen stimulation. The outer surface of the cell becomes more folded, the individual granules coalesce and form channels to the surface through which their contents are released. They lose their typical scrolled and crystalloid appearance and ultimately appear empty or vacuolated. Some granules may reach the surface or even be released apparently intact.

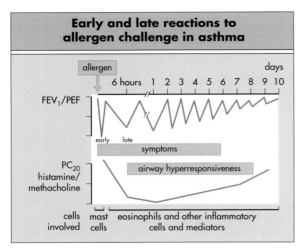

Fig. 3.6. Early and late reactions to allergen challenge in asthma. In the laboratory, patients can be exposed to a single large dose of allergen. This results in an immediate, short-lived decline in lung function as measured by the forced expiratory volume in 1 second (FEV_1) or the peak expiratory flow (PEF). The decline is commonly followed within 6 hours or more by a late-phase reaction. The early reaction is usually reversible by inhaled bronchodilator therapy, but the late reaction is much less readily reversed. Symptoms of asthma may persist for several days, especially at night, and PEF readings may show low early morning values ('morning dipping'). Over the same period, there is an increase in airway responsiveness, as measured by histamine or methacholine challenge tests. Mast cells have a predominant role in the immediate reaction to allergen challenge, but other inflammatory cells and mediators have the predominant role in the prolonged late reaction.

Eosinophils

Other inflammatory cells are believed to be more important than mast cells in chronic asthma. Eosinophils are now known to play an important role in both airway inflammation and AHR. Asthmatic inflammation is characterised by an infiltrate rich in activated eosinophils (**Fig. 3.7**). Eosinophils release several mediators including lipid mediators, cytokines and oxygen radicals, and their granules also contain various toxic basic proteins (**Figs 3.8, 3.9**), the release of which may contribute to the process of epithelial shedding (*see* **Figs 2.4, 2.5, 2.9, 2.11**).

The different stages of eosinophilic inflammation are controlled by specific 'signals'. The initial stage involves adhesion of the eosinophils to the vascular endothelium. Subsequently, eosinophils migrate via gaps in the vascular endothelium (**Fig. 3.10**) into the tissue, where they are primed and activated. These events are co-ordinated by multiple mediators and cytokines.

T lymphocytes

T lymphocytes are present in increased numbers in asthmatic airways and immunological markers show that they are activated. They play an important role in orchestrating and perpetuating the chronic inflammatory response in asthma where they programme the proliferation of a subset of helper T cells (TH2 cells) which release various cytokines (*see* **Fig. 3.11**, page 22).

Airway epithelial cells

Mediators from eosinophils and other cells lead to epithelial shedding, and at this stage the airway epithelial cells themselves may release several important mediators. Epithelial shedding may thus have several consequences:

- Increased airway permeability, which allows easier access of allergens to submucosal structures and greater plasma exudation into the airway lumen (see below).
- Loss of epithelial-derived relaxant factor (EpDRF), which would normally protect against bronchoconstriction.
- Loss of the enzyme neutral endopeptidase (NEP), which would normally degrade bronchoconstrictor peptides.
- Release of cytokines, which may increase the inflammatory response.
- Exposure of sensory nerve endings, which can lead to the activation of neural reflexes.

All these factors tend to lead to airway hyperresponsiveness.

Macrophages

The number of alveolar macrophages is increased in asthma, and they are known to release a wide range of lipid mediators, oxygen radicals and nitric oxide (NO) as well as numerous cytokines. Alveolar macrophages may be activated by a number of mechanisms including a low-affinity IgE receptor, and their involvement in asthma probably helps to determine the type of inflammatory response which develops.

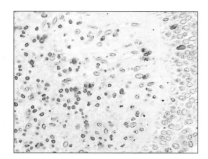

Fig. 3.7. Immunohistochemistry may be used to study cellular infiltration in asthma. In this section of the airway wall from a patient with mild asthma, activated eosinophils are stained red–brown by a technique involving the monoclonal antibody EG_2. Normal airways show no more than a very occasional eosinophil when stained by this technique. The presence of eosinophils is so characteristic of asthma that some have suggested that asthma should be defined as 'eosinophilic bronchitis'.

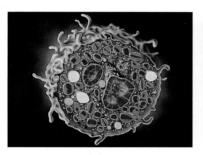

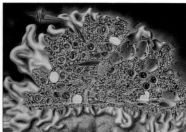

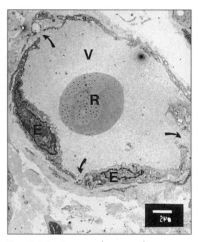

Fig. 3.8. Eosinophil. This artist's representation of a cross section shows the typical appearance of the dormant cell. There are at least four different types of secretory granule within the cell, the most characteristic of which contain a dense crystalline core, surrounded by an amorphous matrix. The granules contain cubic lattice crystals which consist of major basic protein (MBP). The surrounding matrix of the granule contains, amongst other mediators, eosinophil cationic protein (ECP), eosinophil-derived neurotoxin (EDN) and eosinophil peroxidase (EPO). Eosinophils also contain a number of inflammatory mediators, including lipid mediators, oxygen radicals and cytokines.

Fig. 3.9. Secreting eosinophil. This artist's representation shows the cross section of an activated cell. Eosinophils are mobile and flexible, and those in areas of allergic inflammation are usually irregular in shape and in an activated state. Many of the granules are pale and empty in appearance as their contents have been released. This release seems to take place in at least two ways: by fusion with the cell membrane and via 'pores' in the cell surface. The basic proteins released from the granules are intensely toxic to parasites and also damaging to human epithelium. They are thought to contribute to the process of epithelial shedding. The other mediators released have important effects in modulating and perpetuating the inflammatory process.

Fig. 3.10. Gaps in the vascular endothelium in asthma are associated with airway inflammation, and they are the route through which inflammatory cells migrate into the tissues and plasma exudation occurs. This is an electron-microscopic section of a post-capillary venule from the bronchial wall of a patient with asthma. A red blood cell (R) can be seen within the lumen of the venule (V). Prominent gaps (arrowed) can be seen between the endothelial cells (E) of the venule wall.

Other cells

Changes in other cells are also relevant to the mechanisms of asthma and the response of asthma to therapy. Dendritic cells and B lymphocytes are involved in the initiation and perpetuation of the inflammatory response. Platelets may release mediators which influence eosinophil function. The number of β_2-adrenoreceptors on smooth muscle cells is variable, and may be increased by steroid therapy. Fibroblast activity is affected by mediators released by epithelial cells and macrophages. Endothelial cell function is influenced by cytokines released by T lymphocytes.

Cytokine networks in asthma

Cytokines are important mediators of chronic inflammation, and the network of cytokines determines the nature of the inflammatory response. A current view of the most important cytokine networks is shown in **Fig. 3.11**.

OTHER IMPORTANT MECHANISMS IN ASTHMA

Plasma exudation

Microvascular leakage in asthmatic airways may be triggered by many inflammatory mediators and have several consequences. Plasma exudation occurs through gaps in the endothelium of the microvasculature (**Fig. 3.10**) into the interstitium of the airway wall, where it is associated with oedema (**Fig. 3.12**). Plasma proteins then pass between epithelial cells, exacerbating epithelial shedding. Plasma exudation into the lumen of the airways leads to mucus plugging, decreased mucociliary clearance, and the release of kinins and complement fragments, all of which contribute to airway hyperresponsiveness.

When epithelial shedding is accompanied by plasma exudation, it may be followed by the rapid formation of a fibrin gel on the surface of the denuded epithelium. This leads to further airway narrowing, but it may have a protective function, as it lessens airway permeability, and rapid restitution of normal epithelium may take place beneath the fibrin gel.

Neurogenic mechanisms

Neurogenic mechanisms probably play an important part in producing or amplifying symptoms in asthma. Inflammatory mediators may promote the release of neurotransmitters from airway nerves, and some neurotransmitters, especially neuropeptides, may also have amplifying effects on the inflammatory response (**Fig 3.13**).

EFFECTS OF INFLAMMATION IN ASTHMA

It is important to distinguish the acute and chronic inflammatory changes in asthma (**Fig. 3.14**). The acute changes are potentially reversible, and they usually resolve completely with effective anti-inflammatory therapy. By contrast, the chronic inflammatory processes lead to structural changes in the airways in asthma ('remodelling'), which may prove irreversible. This understanding provides the fundamental rationale for the concept of early intervention with effective anti-inflammatory therapy in asthma.

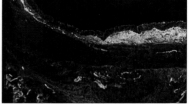

Fig. 3.12. **Plasma exudation** is one of the earliest signs of inflammation in the respiratory mucosa. This sample was obtained 30 seconds after allergen challenge in a guinea pig, and it shows dense plasma exudation in the extravascular tissue of the lamina propria region (demonstrated by epipolarisation microscopy with a colloidal gold plasma tracer). This leads to oedema and to exudation of plasma into the lumen; it may also contribute to epithelial shedding. Plasma exudation can be blocked by prior treatment with a topical steroid.

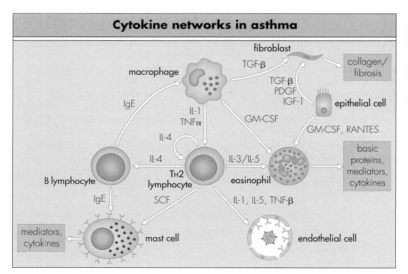

Fig. 3.11. **Cytokine networks in asthma** determine the nature of the inflammatory response and it is likely that many cytokines play important roles in the pathogenesis of asthma. The best established roles are shown here. (IL = interleukin; GM-CSF = granulocyte–macrophage colony stimulating factor; TNF = tumour necrosis factor; TGF = transforming growth factor; RANTES = released by activated normal T cells, expressed and secreted; PDGF = platelet derived growth factor; IGF = insulin-like growth factor; SCF = stem cell factor.)

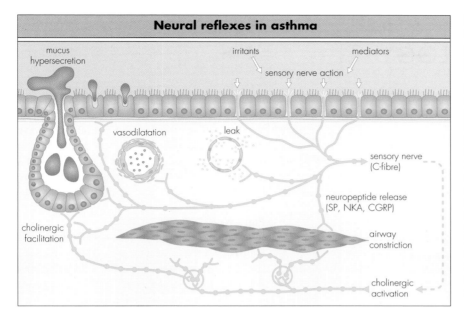

Neural reflexes in asthma

mucus hypersecretion

irritants

mediators

sensory nerve action

vasodilatation

leak

sensory nerve (C-fibre)

neuropeptide release (SP, NKA, CGRP)

cholinergic facilitation

airway constriction

cholinergic activation

Fig. 3.13. Neural reflexes in asthma. Sensory nerves probably play an important role in asthmatic inflammation. They can be sensitised by the products of inflammation and activated by inhaled irritants and by mediators such as bradykinin. Neural reflexes may lead to cholinergic bronchoconstriction and to the release of neuropeptides, such as substance P (SP), neurokinin A (NKA) and calcitonin gene-related peptide (CGRP), which act on target cells in the airways to increase inflammation. Neuropeptides may cause vasodilatation, microvascular leakage and mucus secretion, as well as smooth muscle contraction.

THERAPEUTIC IMPLICATIONS OF ASTHMA MECHANISMS

The balance of mechanisms undoubtedly differs in different patients with asthma, but a number of different cell types and multiple mediators are always involved. There is no evidence that blockade of a single mediator can be effective in controlling and preventing the progression of asthma, although much research has been directed towards this end.

Cromones act by stabilising the mast cell membrane, preventing antigen-induced release of histamine and other mediators. Sodium cromoglycate (cromolyn) and nedocromil sodium may have an additional effect by inhibiting the activation of sensory C fibres in the airway wall.

β_2-agonists act mainly by relaxing smooth muscle, They also have mast cell stabilising effects, which may be beneficial in blocking the early reaction to allergens and other stimuli, such as exercise, but which are rapidly diminished by tachyphylaxis with continuous therapy. It is unlikely that β_2-agonists have useful clinical effects on chronic inflammation in asthma.

Steroids, by contrast, are very effective against the chronic inflammatory process, and this effect leads to a fall in AHR and to control of asthma symptoms. The efficacy of inhaled steroid therapy in asthma probably results from the fact that steroids do not affect a single mediator; they have a multiplicity of actions on the cells and cytokines involved in the inflammatory

process. Their intracellular effects on messenger RNA (mRNA) production lead to the down-regulation of the production and release of a range of pro-inflammatory cytokines and other proteins, and to the up-regulation of a range of anti-inflammatory mediators. This generalised anti-inflammatory effect is currently the most effective approach to therapy for most patients with asthma (see page 98).

Changes in acute and chronic asthma

Acute asthma
- Airway constriction
- Vasodilatation
- Microvascular leakage resulting in oedema and plasma exudation into the airway lumen
- Mucus hypersecretion
- Airway hyperresponsiveness

Chronic asthma
- Thickening of the basement membrane and fibrosis under the airway epithelium
- New blood vessel formation
- Thickening of the smooth muscle layer of the airway epithelium (hypertrophy/hyperplasia)
- Hyperplasia of submucosal glands and goblet cells

Fig. 3.14. The contrast between the reversible inflammatory processes involved in acute asthma, and the 'remodelling' processes associated with inflammation in chronic asthma.

4 PHYSIOLOGY

INTRODUCTION

The branching structure of the airways produces a marked increase in the overall cross-sectional area on moving out through the divisions towards the periphery of the lung. The area increases from 2 cm² at the trachea to forty times this at the terminal bronchioles and increases nearly four times again after three divisions of respiratory bronchioles (**Figs 4.1, 4.2**). Consequently airflow slows on moving out through the lung and at the level of the respiratory bronchioles gas movement is by diffusion.

The great increase in cross-sectional area of the airways also means that, at a peripheral level, a large amount of damage has to occur to cause significant symptoms. In contrast, narrowing of the larger airways will produce symptoms early, although the site of the narrowing may not be recognised (*see* page 47). Asthma is a diffuse disease affecting airways throughout the lung. However, there are regional differences in ventilation as shown by the patchy changes in ventilation scans (**Fig. 4.3**).

If flow is laminar then resistance is inversely related to the fourth power of the radius so that resistance increases 16 times if the radius of an airway is halved. This makes small degrees of airway narrowing or bronchodilatation very important. In fact, laminar flow probably occurs mainly in very small airways. In larger airways flow is mostly transitional between laminar and turbulent flow.

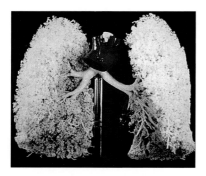

Fig. 4.1. Dissolution cast of the airways. The airways have been injected with resin and the lung structure subsequently dissolved away. This shows the extensive division of the airways producing a huge increase in airway number, reduction in calibre of individual airways but great increase in the overall cross-sectional diameter. The larger airways (trachea, bronchi) are supported by cartilage, the middle size (1–2 mm diameter) have a substantial smooth muscle content, while airways below 1 mm diameter have less smooth muscle so that airway narrowing is more dependent on mucosal thickening than smooth muscle contraction.

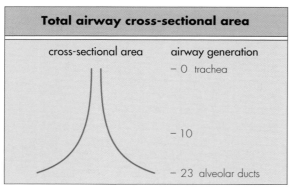

Fig. 4.2. Diagrammatic representation of the total airway cross-sectional area moving out through the bronchial tree. The great increase in cross-sectional diameter means that speed of airflow slows markedly moving out into the lung, peripherally there is no mass flow and gas exchange is achieved by diffusion.

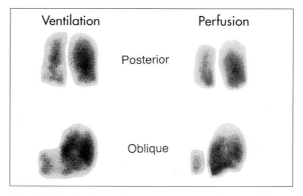

Fig. 4.3. Ventilation perfusion scan in an asthmatic. The airway narrowing in asthma is not uniform, producing patchy abnormalities in distribution of ventilation. There are similar matched reductions in perfusion. This contrasts to the picture in pulmonary embolism, where reduced perfusion is not matched by a reduction in ventilation.

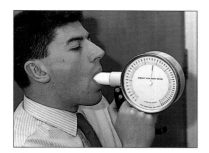

Fig. 4.4. Wright's peak flow meter. This is the standard peak expiratory flow meter used in most respiratory function laboratories. After a maximal inspiration the patient is asked to make a short sharp expiration as fast as possible. The meter registers the maximal flow sustained for 10 milliseconds. Few patients are unable to carry out this test. The procedure is repeated to obtain three technically satisfactory blows and the maximum value taken. In asthma the deep inspiration may trigger airway narrowing, resulting in a decline in peak flow through the three manoeuvres.

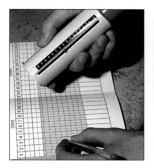

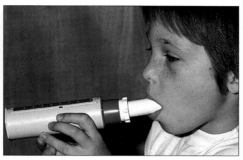

Figs 4.5, 4.6. Portable peak flow meter. A number of cheap portable devices are available for the measurement of peak flow rate at home. They can be used to establish a diagnosis of asthma, to assess the effects of treatment and to monitor control. The results should be monitored and used as part of a written individual management plan for the control of a patient's asthma.

MEASUREMENT OF RESPIRATORY FUNCTION

Narrowing of the airways in asthma is produced by smooth muscle contraction, thickening of the airway wall and mucus in the airways (*see* **Fig. 2.13**). Intrapulmonary airways narrow more on expiration, but both inspiratory and expiratory flows are limited in asthma. Most respiratory function measurements are made on forced expiration. The simplest test of respiratory function is a brief forced expiratory manoeuvre to obtain a peak expiratory flow (PEF). This measures the maximum peak flow maintained for at least 10 msec and requires a brief, forced expiration from a full inspiration. The standard device for PEF measurement is the Wright peak flow meter (**Fig. 4.4**). Peak flow measurements are used in the assessment of acute asthma, the measurement of response to therapy and for repeated measurements in the assessment of the pattern of asthma in an individual patient. Home recordings are possible with one of a variety of cheap, portable devices (**Figs 4.5, 4.6**). Peak flow rate varies according to age, height and sex; tables and figures of normal values are available (**Fig. 4.7**).

The calibration on most commercially available peak flow meters is not linearly related to the flow generated in a pattern similar to expiratory flow. In North America different scales which meet NHLBI standards are available. In practice, as long as a patient uses a similar device consistently and the same device as any doctor making an assessment in a clinic or hospital there should be no problems, since it is the pattern and the trends which are most important.

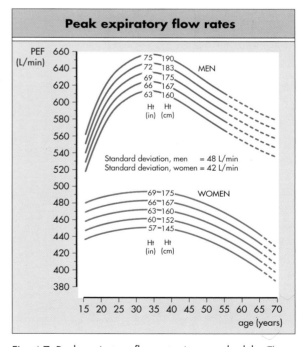

Fig. 4.7. Peak expiratory flow rates in normal adults. The chart shows the normal values for peak flow rate in men and women between 15 and 70 years. The confidence intervals around the normal values are 100 L/min in men and 85 L/min in women.

Spirometry (**Fig. 4.8**) allows the measurement of forced vital capacity (FVC) and timed measurements of volume such as the forced expiratory volume in the first second (FEV_1) (**Fig. 4.9**). In the spirogram the PEF is the maximum slope of the volume time trace, but this is easier to appreciate on a plot of flow against volume (**Fig. 4.10**).

In asthma the narrowing of the airways causes an obstructive defect with a reduction in the normal ratio of FEV_1 to FVC. This is expressed as the forced expiratory ratio (FER). As asthma becomes more severe the lung volumes increase and the FVC is reduced also. The overinflation of asthma is largely produced by active contraction of abdominal muscles braking expiration. The higher volumes may be an attempt to widen the airways in the lung and to prevent airway collapse in some areas. The overinflation moves the patient up the pressure–volume curve of the lungs (*see* **Fig. 5.1**). This means that more work is required to take in a given volume on inspiration, breathlessness occurs on inspiration and the vital capacity is restricted.

When the forced expiration is displayed as flow and volume, the volume axis is displayed horizontally (**Fig. 4.10**). As asthma worsens the residual volume increases and the flows drop on the flow–volume curve with dipping of the loop as flow rates at lower lung volumes

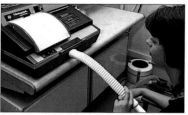

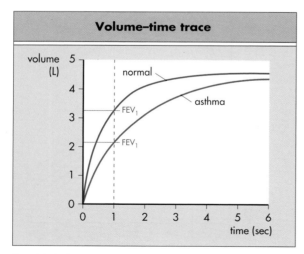

Fig. 4.8. Forced expired vital capacity measurement using a bellows spirometer. A convenient assessment of airflow obstruction is the forced expired vital capacity manoeuvre where the patient takes a maximal inspiration and is then asked to exhale as fast as possible for as long as possible. The volume expired against time is measured and the forced expired volume in one second (FEV_1) can be determined, as can the forced vital capacity (FVC). The ratio of FEV_1/FVC if reduced (less than 80%) suggests airflow obstruction, but each variate can be assessed against predicted values which depend on sex, age, height and ethnic origin. Respiratory function laboratories usually measure FEV_1/FVC using bellows type spirometers, but increasingly smaller turbine or other electronic devices are used.

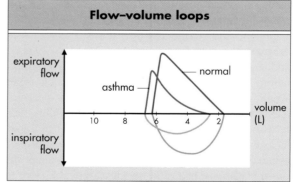

Fig. 4.10. Flow–volume loops. The forced expiratory manoeuvre can also be displayed as flow against volume. Conventionally volume is displayed on the horizontal axis. A maximum inspiratory breath can be included to give the full loop. In asthma both inspiratory flow and expiratory flow are reduced and the residual volume is increased. After a bronchodilator the expiratory and inspiratory flows should increase and residual volume and total lung capacity may decrease. Changes in lung volume may produce symptomatic improvement with minimal increases in FEV_1 or FVC.

Fig. 4.9. Volume–time trace. Spirometers or pneumotachographs are used to produce a volume time trace of forced expiration. In normal subjects the vital capacity is expelled in less than 5 seconds and around 75% of this is produced in the first second (FEV_1). In asthma the FEV_1 is reduced to a greater extent than any reduction in FVC (forced vital capacity).

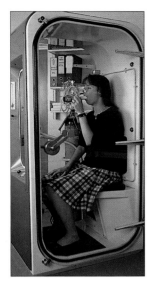

Fig. 4.11. Body plethysmograph. Airways resistance and thoracic gas volume can be measured in the body plethysmograph. Measurements of lung volume may differ from those achieved by helium dilution techniques. The plethysmograph volume estimations include all gas subject to alveolar pressures even if it is not in communication with the airways, e.g. pneumothorax, trapped gas. Helium dilution only includes gas which can communicate with the inspired air within a reasonable time.

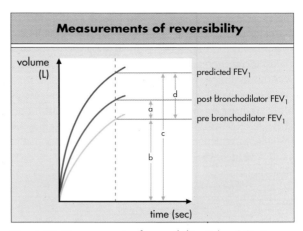

Fig. 4.12. Measurements of reversibility. Reversibility in a measurement such as FEV_1 can be expressed as absolute change (a), percentage change (100 x a/b), percentage predicted (100 x a/c) or percentage possible (100 x a/d).

decline (forced expiratory flow (FEF) at 25% or 50% vital capacity). The dipping of the flows at lower lung volumes may reflect changes in the small airways of the lung. An inspiratory limb can be measured also. The normal inspiratory loop looks like a semicircle, but the flows are progressively lowered as asthma worsens.

The typical flow volume loop in asthma is distinct from that in emphysema or in large airway narrowing (*see* page 47).

Airway narrowing can also be measured as airways resistance. This will vary with the degree of inflation and can be expressed as specific airways resistance where the resistance value is divided by lung volume at which it is performed. Conductance is the reciprocal of resistance and can also be standardised for lung volume as specific conductance. The airways resistance is measured in a body plethysmograph (**Fig. 4.11**).

REVERSIBILITY

Reversibility of airflow obstruction is assessed after administration of a bronchodilator. Short acting β_2-agonists are used in a dose such as 200 µg salbutamol or 500 µg terbutaline. Occasionally responses to larger doses, such as those given from a nebuliser, or responses to anticholinergic agents, such as ipratropium bromide, are tested. β-Agonist responses are measured at 20–30 minutes and anticholinergic responses at 40–60 minutes.

Reversibility is used as part of the usual definitions of asthma, but the degree of reversibility is often not stated. Reversibility can be expressed in various ways.

Percentage of baseline is the commonest form but, with a low starting level, 15–20% of baseline may be well within the variability of the test. Other possibilities are to report the absolute change or express change as a percentage of the difference between the starting level and that predicted. The 95% confidence intervals of the tests mean that changes of 70 L/min in PEF, 200 mL in FEV_1 and 350 mL in FVC are needed to be sure that a change is significant. These criteria should be added to any requirement for a percentage change in baseline (**Fig. 4.12**).

AIRWAY HYPERRESPONSIVENESS (AHR)

Apart from reversibility of airflow obstruction, the other functional characteristic of asthma is increased responsiveness of the airways. The inflamed mucosa of the airways is abnormally sensitive to a variety of non-allergic and non-sensitising stimuli, including exercise, cold air, dust, smoke and chemical stimuli such as methacholine or histamine. Most asthmatics show a response to abnormally low levels of challenging agent and the level of responsiveness is related to the severity of the asthma and the need for treatment. Atopic subjects with hayfever but not asthma often show an intermediate level of responsiveness which increases further in more severe asthma (**Fig. 4.13**). The responsiveness is expressed as the *concentration* of the provoking agent required to decrease FEV_1 by a set percentage, e.g. 20% (the PC_{20}), or specific airways conductance by 35%. Alternatively, the responsiveness may be expressed as the *dose* of agent required to decrease the FEV_1 by a set percentage (e.g. the PD_{20} – **Fig. 4.14**). Normal subjects may sometimes show increased responsiveness, but asthmatics with normal airway responsiveness are unusual.

Responsiveness in patients with asthma increases after viral upper respiratory tract infections and after allergen exposure, often for several days. This may be the way in which such events lead to loss of control in asthma (**Fig. 4.15**).

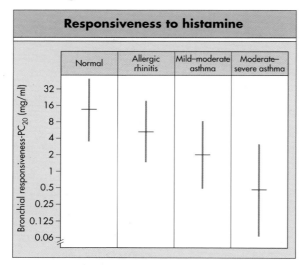

Fig. 4.13. **Responsiveness to histamine** in normals, rhinitics and patients with different severities of asthma. Although there is a great deal of overlap there is a trend for increasing bronchial responsiveness moving from normals through patients with hayfever to various grades of severity of asthma.

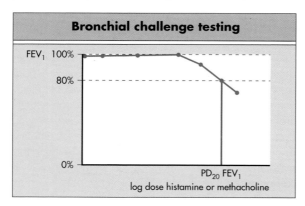

Fig. 4.14. **Bronchial challenge testing** with inhaled histamine Doubling doses are given and FEV_1 measured after each dose. The cumulative dose which produces a 20% drop in FEV_1 or a 35% reduction in specific airways conductance is estimated by linear interpolation from the two surrounding values. Challenge tests with allergen may also provoke late reactions (*see* **Fig. 3.6**) but these are not seen with histamine or methacholine.

Responsiveness to bronchoconstrictor challenges can be reduced by avoidance of exposure to a known allergen, e.g. house dust mite, or by use of a regular prophylactic agent such as an inhaled steroid. Bronchodilators reduce responsiveness, but only for a short time, usually less than the length of their bronchodilator action.

Responsiveness is not often measured in the routine investigation of asthma in the UK. In some other countries it is a more commonly used laboratory test in asthmatics. It is certainly useful in the investigation of occupational asthma or in difficult asthma, such as that presenting as chronic cough; it is commonly measured in trials of drug therapy in asthma, where it may serve as a surrogate marker for inflammation of the airways.

BLOOD GASES

In asthma there is a drop in PaO_2 as ventilation and perfusion matching is disturbed. This is compensated for by an increase in alveolar ventilation and consequently a decrease in $PaCO_2$. In acute asthma this can be used as a guide to progress since a normal or high level of $PaCO_2$ suggests that the patient is tiring and that support of ventilation will be necessary if intensive treatment fails to produce improvement. If $PaCO_2$ is initially low then oxygenation can be followed by monitoring oxygen saturation with a pulse oximeter, unless there is a deterioration in the clinical condition when blood gases should be repeated.

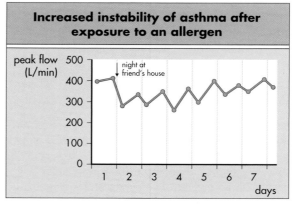

Fig. 4.15. **Increased instability of asthma** after exposure to an allergen. This graph shows the increased diurnal variation in peak flow which followed an exposure to house dust mite when a 15-year-old girl visited a friend's house for one night.

5 | CLINICAL FEATURES

SYMPTOMS

Shortness of breath

Shortness of breath is the commonest symptom of asthma. It is a response to the increase in work of breathing associated with narrowing of the airways and overinflation of the chest. The measurements performed to quantify the severity of asthma are usually forced expiratory manoeuvres. However, patients in an acute asthmatic attack are more likely to complain of difficulties with inspiration than expiration. This is because of the overinflation associated with acute asthma. The increase in volume means that larger transthoracic pressures are necessary to produce a given volume change (**Fig. 5.1**).

In a severe attack of asthma, shortness of breath can be a frightening symptom which makes the patient very anxious. It is important that such anxiety is recognised as a secondary phenomenon and that treatment is directed at the underlying airflow obstruction and not at the anxiety itself.

The hallmark of asthma is the variability in the degree of airflow obstruction. This is reflected in the symptoms of variable breathlessness. Increases in breathlessness may be associated with identifiable triggers of asthma (*see* Chapter 6), such as allergens or cold air, or part of the spontaneous diurnal variation in airway calibre which is accentuated markedly in asthmatics (**Fig. 5.2**). Questioning on nocturnal symptoms is a very important part of taking the history in asthma; waking at night with breathlessness is a sign of poor disease control.

The relationship between symptoms and objective measurements of airway calibre is good in most patients, but a substantial minority have poor perception of the state of their asthma. There is likely to be an increased risk that such patients can deteriorate into an acute exacerbation without warning. Objective records of peak flow may be particularly important in this group to allow them to be aware of a deterioration and to abort an acute attack by an increase in treatment. There is some evidence that patients who develop severe, life-threatening exacerbations are more likely to fall into this group of poor perceivers of the state of their asthma (**Fig. 5.3**).

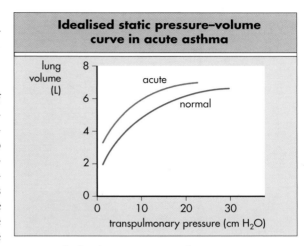

Fig. 5.1. Idealised static pressure–volume curve in acute asthma. Functional residual capacity may be increased in acute asthma; because of the shape of the pressure–volume curve, more pressure needs to be generated to produce a given volume of inspiration.

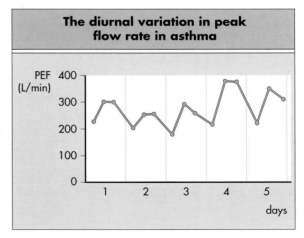

Fig. 5.2. The diurnal variation in peak flow in asthma results in lowest peak flow rates in the early hours of the morning. Questions about the quality of sleep and nocturnal awakenings with cough or shortness of breath are important in the clinical history of any asthma patient. An improvement in the overall level of peak flow may take the patient out of the symptomatic range especially during the daytime. Perception of the degree of airways obstruction shows marked variability between individuals.

Occasionally patients may complain of tightness of the chest which can be confused with ischaemic heart disease. The tightness is related to the increased lung volume and careful questioning will distinguish the symptoms.

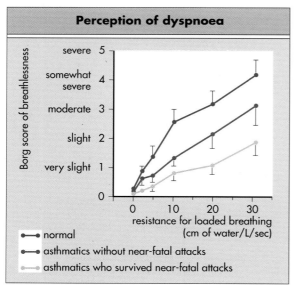

Perception of dyspnoea

Borg score of breathlessness:
- severe 5
- somewhat severe 4
- moderate 3
- slight 2
- very slight 1
- 0

resistance for loaded breathing (cm of water/L/sec): 0 10 20 30

- normal
- asthmatics without near-fatal attacks
- asthmatics who survived near-fatal attacks

Fig. 5.3. Perception of dyspnoea during breathing. In this study, patients who had survived a near-fatal episode of asthma had a reduced sensation of breathlessness when asked to breathe against resistance loading. Hypoxic response was reduced as well. The reduced perception of obstruction and reduced response may identify a vulnerable group of patients who fail to react to deteriorating asthma. (Adapted from Kikuchi et al., N Eng J Med, 1994: **330**; 1329.)

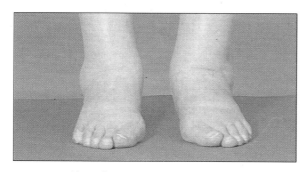

Fig. 5.4. Ankle oedema. Occasionally asthma may present as chronic respiratory failure with hypoxia, pulmonary hypertension and ankle oedema. In these circumstances vigorous treatment of the asthma may result in marked improvements in airflow obstruction and resolution of the cor pulmonale. After such chronic untreated disease complete reversal of airways narrowing to predicted values of airflow is unlikely.

Cough

Cough is a common symptom of asthma. This is likely to reflect the inflammatory change in the wall of the airway. It may even be the sole presenting manifestation of asthma. In studies of previously unexplained chronic cough, asthma is the commonest underlying cause detected on detailed investigation. The diagnosis may be helped by finding increased nonspecific bronchial reactivity to methacholine or histamine, or a symptomatic response to asthma therapy. In some cases a short course of oral corticosteroids may be necessary to settle the cough even in the absence of significant airflow obstruction. Patients who present with cough as the sole manifestation of asthma may later progress to develop airflow obstruction as part of their asthma.

There are hypertrophied mucus glands in the inflamed airways in asthma and the cough may be associated with sputum production. The sputum may be clear or mucoid, or it may be green or yellow. The colour is produced by degenerating white cells which are eosinophils in asthma but neutrophils in the purulent sputum associated with superimposed respiratory infections. The sputum may be particularly sticky and form plugs which are difficult to expectorate and may be teased out to show casts of the airways (*see* **Fig. 2.10**). This is seen most prominently in allergic broncho-pulmonary aspergillosis (ABPA, *see* below). In fatal asthma, obstruction of the airways by plugs is a prominent finding (*see* **Fig. 2.11**).

Presentation as respiratory failure

Occasionally patients may be very insensitive to the effects of their asthma, allowing severe obstruction and hypoxia to develop before seeking any help. Such patients present with right heart failure (**Fig. 5.4**) and severe airflow obstruction. They may be dismissed as having irreversible obstruction, but it is always worth making vigorous efforts to treat the airway narrowing in these patients who are first seen with cor pulmonale.

Irreversible asthma

Although in most cases, particularly in the young, asthma has a large reversible element, a considerable irreversible element may develop in older patients with chronic asthma. It has been shown that the degree of irreversible obstruction in adults is related

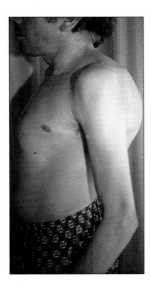

Fig. 5.5. Kyphoscoliosis and overexpansion in an adult asthmatic with a history of severe asthma, with recurrent hospital admissions. Such deformity is only associated with chronic severe asthma through childhood.

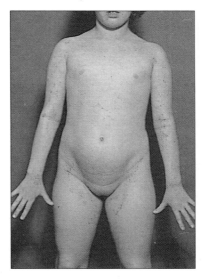

Fig. 5.6. Flexural eczema. Eczema is a common accompaniment of the atopic state. Anecdotally many asthmatics with chronic eczema find that the clinical state of their asthma is negatively correlated with the condition of their eczema.

to the duration and severity of earlier disease. The irreversibility is associated with pathological damage in the airway, with fibrosis under the basement membrane (see Chapter 2). It is hoped that more vigorous treatment of the airway inflammation early in asthma may limit the damage to the airway wall and reduce the risk of irreversible obstruction later. There is some evidence from the trials of early intervention with inhaled steroids that this may be so (*see* **Figs 15.6, 15.7**).

SIGNS

Overinflation

In an acute attack of asthma and in chronic uncontrolled asthma, lung volume is increased. This may be detectable as overinflation of the chest on examination (**Fig. 5.5**).

Wheeze

Wheezing is a characteristic feature of asthma caused by airflow through narrowed airways. The wheezing is mainly expiratory because intrathoracic airways are narrower in expiration, but it may also be heard during inspiration. There are multiple wheezes at different pitches because airways of different calibre are narrowed. This is in contrast to the monophonic wheeze of a large airway obstruction which is often as loud or louder on inspiration.

ASSOCIATED CONDITIONS

Atopic eczema

The atopic state is associated with allergic rhinitis and with eczema as well as asthma. Evidence of these conditions may be present at the time of examination. The distribution of eczema varies with age but is often flexural (**Fig. 5.6**).

Rhinitis and nasal polyposis

Rhinitis may be seasonal from sensitivity to pollens or fungal spores or may be related to other allergens such as house dust mite or animals. Nasal polyps may also be associated with asthma (**Fig. 5.7**), especially in older patients with aspirin sensitivity (*see* page 125).

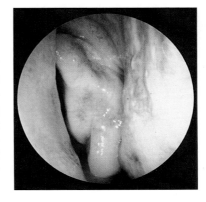

Fig. 5.7. Nasal polyposis is a relatively frequent accompaniment of asthma and is particularly common in adult asthmatics with sensitivity to aspirin. Polyps may be reduced in size by topical or oral steroid therapy.

Allergic broncho-pulmonary aspergillosis

Aspergillus fungal spores are ubiquitous (**Fig. 5.8**). Higher counts are associated with decaying vegetation such as compost heaps and with disturbance of old buildings or the ground, as at demolition sites. Aspergillus is associated with a number of pulmonary conditions including fungal balls (mycetomas) in lung cavities, invasive aspergillosis in immunosuppressed patients, asthma from sensitivity to aspergillus spores and allergic broncho-pulmonary aspergillosis (ABPA). In ABPA there is an allergic response to *Aspergillus fumigatus* spores in the airway. This leads to an IgE-mediated reaction in the wall and the lumen of the airway. Rubbery plugs made up of mixtures of mucus, aspergillus hyphae and eosinophils may obstruct the airway (**Figs 5.9, 5.10**). This leads to lobar or segmental collapse (**Figs 5.11, 5.12**) and to damage to the adjacent airway wall causing proximal bronchiectasis.

The patient often gives a history of expectoration of rubbery brownish plugs and examination of these will show fungal hyphae and eosinophils. The eosinophil count in the blood is raised during exacerbations of ABPA. The skin prick test for aspergillus is positive and specific IgE against *Aspergillus fumigatus* can be detected in the blood. The total IgE is usually raised.

Treatment is with corticosteroids to suppress an attack. Oral steroids have been used to reduce the frequency of exacerbations of ABPA and, more recently, itraconazole has been used for the same purpose.

Allergic granulomatosis

Allergic granulomatosis (Churg–Strauss syndrome) is covered on page 48.

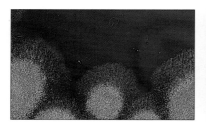

Fig. 5.8. Fruiting bodies of the aspergillus fungus growing in culture. These form in the tissues if the growth of aspergillus is profuse. Culture of sputum plugs should be performed if allergic broncho-pulmonary aspergillosis is suspected.

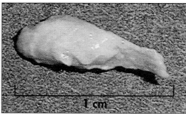

Fig. 5.9. Typical sputum plug of allergic broncho-pulmonary aspergillosis. These are usually brownish and firm or rubbery. On microscopy or culture they show *Aspergillus*. This plug was aspirated at fibreoptic bronchoscopy in a patient with segmental collapse on the chest radiograph.

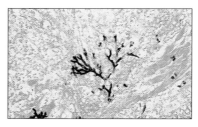

Fig. 5.10. *Aspergillus fumigatus* in a sputum plug. The fungal hyphae show up very well with this Grocott stain. The typical hyphal branching structure at approximately 45° is characteristic.

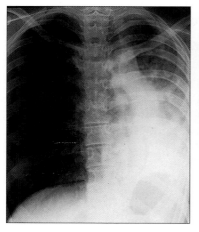

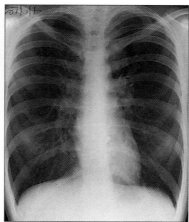

Figs 5.11 and 5.12. Lobar collapse in a case of allergic broncho-pulmonary aspergillosis. The left lower lobe and possibly the lingula have collapsed with deviation of the mediastinum to the left side (left). Re-expansion of the lobe after physiotherapy and bronchodilators (right) resulted in expectoration of sticky mucus plugs. Prolonged courses of oral steroids may be necessary to maintain the patient free of exacerbations.

6 INDUCERS AND TRIGGERS

Inducers of asthma act mainly by inducing airway inflammation. It is possible that some symptoms of asthma, including cough and chest tightness, may be directly associated with the presence of airway inflammation, but the classical symptoms of wheezing and dyspnoea are believed to result from the airway hyperresponsiveness (AHR) which accompanies airway inflammation. *Triggers* of asthma are factors which cause airway smooth muscle contraction and asthma symptoms on a background of pre-existing AHR. The relationship between inducers and triggers is further discussed in Chapter 3 and summarised in **Fig. 6.1**.

It seems likely that a single inducer, combined with a genetic predisposition, is sufficient to initiate asthma. The atopic nature of many asthmatics is, however, often associated with a tendency to form IgE antibodies against a range of common inhaled allergens, and viral infections in infancy or environmental factors may also play a role; so multiple inducers may contribute to asthma in many patients. The true prevention of asthma requires the prevention of this induction process, but this is not yet feasible.

Once asthma is established, the associated AHR makes most patients sensitive to a wide range of triggers, so avoidance of provoking factors alone is usually an inadequate strategy for the control of asthma. A small number of patients with asthma respond mainly to a single trigger, however, in the same way as patients with seasonal rhinitis may respond only to a single type of pollen. It is important to explore this possibility, since occasionally avoidance of, or even desensitisation to, a provoking allergen may be a possible alternative to long-term suppression or prevention of asthma by drug therapy.

ALLERGENS

Allergens are believed to be of fundamental importance in most patients with asthma, and they often have an important role as both inducers and triggers. The most important source of allergen worldwide is probably the dust mite, and the increase in dust mite populations which accompanies urban living may be the major explanation

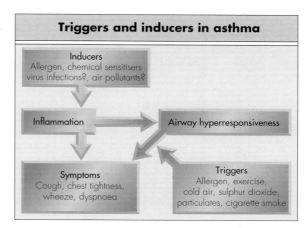

Fig. 6.1. The relationship between inducers and triggers in the provocation of symptoms in asthma.

for the increasing worldwide prevalence of asthma. Other allergens are also important in many patients.

Dust mite

The house dust mite, *Dermatophagoides pteronyssinus* (also *D. farinae*), feeds on shed human skin scales and is found in most samples of house dust, especially in mattresses and soft furnishings in bedrooms. The allergen is present in the faeces of the mite, which can be easily aerosolised to a size which is deposited in the lower respiratory tract. Mites (**Fig. 6.2**) are most abundant in warm humid conditions and proliferate in autumn. The gradual change to centrally heated houses with warm bedrooms from the more austere conditions of 20–40 years ago has increased the numbers of mites in bedrooms. This exposes infants to a heavy antigen load early in life and may have contributed to the rise in the prevalence of asthma.

Contact with dust mites or a lowering in their numbers can be achieved by a number of methods (**Fig. 6.3**). Although these precautions reduce allergen load, they only have a significant effect on the control of asthma if they are done regularly and vigorously. This may be difficult to achieve in practice.

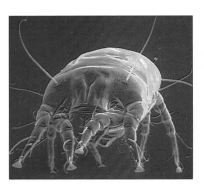

Fig. 6.2. House dust mite (*Dermato-phagoides pteronyssinus*). Scanning electron micrograph of a house dust mite. Fragments of the house dust mite faeces are aerosolysed and inhaled into the airways.

Dust mite control measures	
Barrier methods	Mattress and bedding covers – trap and limit contact with mites. Allow efficient dust removal
Regular vacuum cleaning of carpets, soft furnishings and mattress	Limits dust and the mite population
Chemicals	Acaricides kill mites, but are ineffective when used alone. Fungicides may remove essential fungal foodstuff for the mites. Only really effective on carpets
Temperature	Very low temperatures kill mites (use liquid nitrogen or freeze bedding, etc. – usually impracticable). High temperature, e.g. exposure of carpets to sunlight, kills mites
Humidity	Lower humidity leads to lower mite populations
Spartan furnishings	Removal of carpets, upholstery, etc. removes mite reservoirs and allows easy cleaning

Fig. 6.3. Some methods which can be used to avoid contact with house dust mites or limit their numbers.

Allergenic pollens in Europe	
Region	Allergenic airborne pollens
Arctic	Birch
Central	Deciduous forest trees, birch, grasses
Mediterranean	*Parietaria*, olive trees, cypress, grasses
Eastern	Grasses, mugwort, ragweed
Mountain	Grasses, trees

Fig. 6.4. The principal airborne pollens of relevance to respiratory allergy in the main vegetational zones of Europe.

Pollens

For a plant pollen to cause allergy, it must be allergenic and airborne in large quantities for some time. Many plants worldwide meet these criteria and are responsible for *pollinosis* (asthma and/or allergic rhinitis and conjunctivitis).

In Europe, the distribution of airborne pollen can be related to five different vegetational areas (**Fig. 6.4**), and there are similar differences in pollen distribution on other continents such as North America. The most widely distributed pollens of clinical importance are those of grasses (**Fig. 6.5**), but birch pollen (**Fig. 6.6**) is an important allergen in the Nordic countries, *Parietaria* and olive tree pollens are responsible for

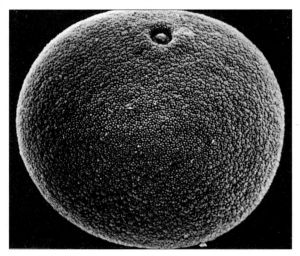

Fig. 6.5. Grass pollen. The prevalent grass pollens vary with the country and area. The grains can be broken up by changes in pressure and humidity and this may increase their ability to enter the tracheo-bronchial tree. This may occur during thunderstorms and result in increased asthma presentations. Otherwise the pollen grains are released at a reasonably predictable time each year.

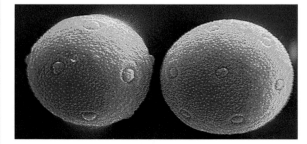

Fig. 6.6. Birch pollen. Tree pollens may have a different time of release from most grasses. Birch pollination is in May. There is cross-reaction between birch and alder, oak, hazel and hornbeam pollens.

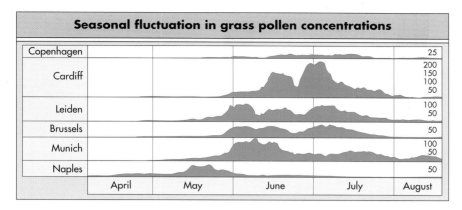

Fig. 6.7. Seasonal fluctuation in grass pollen concentrations at six different sites in Europe (mean values for 1982–86).

many cases of pollinosis in the Mediterranean regions, and weed pollens, especially ragweed, are particularly important in the USA. Cross-reactivity between different pollens (e.g. related grasses or trees) is quite common.

The timing of the pollen season for a single species of grass varies from one region to another (**Fig. 6.7**), and similar variations are seen in the timing of the pollen seasons for other plants. This can result in unexpected symptoms in a patient with known pollinosis who travels from his own region, where the provoking pollen is out of season, to a region where the pollen is in season. It also provides opportunities for pollen avoidance by travel in the appropriate season, though this is rarely a practical possibility for most patients.

Most pollen grains are around 10 µm in diameter. It is easy for them to reach the conjunctiva and the nasal mucosa, causing allergic conjunctivitis and rhinitis, but few particles of this size reach the lower respiratory tract. They may be disrupted, sometimes by climatic change, to produce smaller particles which can then enter the lower respiratory tract and induce asthma. This may be the mechanism for the increase in asthma problems found at the time of some thunderstorms (**Fig. 6.8**).

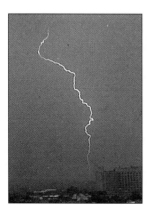

Fig. 6.8. Thunderstorms have been associated with sudden increases in acute severe asthma and asthma mortality in Spain and the UK. This is believed to be the result of the lysis of pollen or other allergen particles into smaller particles which can penetrate into the small airways. Similar increases in asthma symptoms during severe winds have been reported in the USA.

Fungi

Fungal spores, such as those from *Alternaria*, which are plentiful in the late summer and autumn in many countries, are another cause of asthma in some patients. Other moulds such as *Aspergillus* and *Penicillium* may also cause asthma, and these are potentially perennial, as they can occur in damp buildings or stored foodstuffs.

Pets

Almost all furry or feathered pets may cause asthma. Cats are a particularly common cause (*see* **Fig. 16.19**). The allergens may come from skin dander, dried saliva, urine or other products, or as particles from the fur or feathers. The sensitivity may be limited to one species or be more widespread. Anyone who has the tendency to produce IgE to a species of animal is likely to have problems with other pets if they are in close contact and thus given the opportunity to build up their sensitivity. This means that asthmatics should avoid contact with such animals, and those with an atopic history or family should also avoid these pets. In some circumstances the sensitivity may be less obvious; allergens from a horse or other animal may be brought in to the house on clothing or equipment (**Fig. 6.9**).

Food and drink

Intolerance to food and drink is claimed quite frequently in asthma, but relatively few reactions are true allergic responses dependent on specific IgE. True allergic reactions may include urticaria, gastrointestinal disturbances and even anaphylactic shock, particularly to food constituents such as peanuts or shellfish. Other reactions to food are dependent on additives or colouring agents

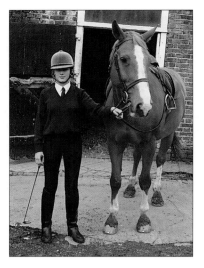

Fig. 6.9. Most animals with fur, hair or feathers can be a trigger for asthma. Contact with allergens from animals can occur in the home or outside. Allergens may also be brought home on clothing to affect other members of the family. The 40-year-old father of this girl had a recurrence of his childhood asthma occurring only at weekends. Skin tests showed a positive response to house dust mite and horse dander. When the daughter changed at the stables after riding and brought her clothes home in a plastic bag the father's asthma resolved.

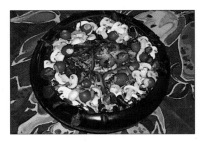

Fig. 6.10. Food allergy. Mixed dishes may make identification of the specific allergen difficult. In a mixed salad many ingredients may be included. Dressings added to the salad may provide a further source. In patients allergic to peanuts small quantities encountered in this way may produce severe reactions.

such as the orange/yellow colouring tartrazine, other azo dyes and benzoate preservatives. Tartrazine is used as a colouring agent in some drugs as well as in foodstuffs.

Sulphur dioxide is used as a preservative in fruit juices and other soft drinks and can provoke asthma in low concentrations. Patients often associate alcoholic drinks with worsening of their asthma; this may be specific to one sort of drink and probably results from constituents other than the alcohol itself.

Sensitivity to food can often be determined from a carefully taken history, but the undeclared presence of substances such as peanuts in prepared foods may make both diagnosis and subsequent avoidance difficult (**Fig. 6.10**). Skin tests and blood tests are rarely helpful in the diagnosis of food allergy, but any diagnostic challenge for asthma should be performed only under carefully controlled conditions.

Drugs

Drugs should always be considered as a possible cause for asthma (**Fig.6.11**). These include drugs bought over the counter (e.g. aspirin), prescribed for another condition (e.g. β-blockers), or even an adverse effect of drugs prescribed for asthma.

β-blockers

No β-blockers are selective enough to be used in asthma, although it may be easier to reverse the effects of the more β_1-selective agents. A history of asthma should be sought in all patients where β-blockers are

considered. Even β-blocker eye drops used for glaucoma have been associated with severe bronchospasm and even death from asthma.

Aspirin

Around 5% of adults give a history of sensitivity to aspirin. On formal testing another 25% may show evidence of increased airway narrowing after aspirin exposure. Chronic exposure may lead to nasal blockage and nasal polyps (*see* **Fig. 5.7**). The problems with aspirin occur also with the non-steroidal anti-inflammatory drugs and seem to result from excessive production of leukotrienes. Usual management is to avoid all such agents, although oral desensitisation may prove possible in experienced hands.

ACE inhibitors

Angiotensin converting enzyme inhibitors cause a cough in around 5% of recipients. This is thought to be through

Drugs which may provoke asthma
• All β-blockers (even 'selective' including eye drops)
• Aspirin
• Non-steroidal anti-inflammatory drugs
• Penicillins
• Inhaled therapy, including asthma therapy
• Angiotensin converting enzyme inhibitors

Fig. 6.11. Drugs which may provoke asthma.

their inhibition of the metabolism of other kinins as well as angiotensin converting enzyme. True asthma is a much rarer complication.

Inhaled therapy

Inhaled therapy may cause 'paradoxical' bronchoconstriction in some patients; this is usually a side-effect of the propellant or other additives in the inhaled preparation, and is rare when pure dry-powder preparations are used. With bronchodilator therapy, any irritant effect is usually masked by the therapeutic effect. Nebuliser solutions can produce problems if they contain preservatives or if they are hypotonic. Reactions to the bromide constituent of anticholinergic drugs and to hydrocortisone preparations are seen occasionally.

OCCUPATIONS

Occupational asthma is asthma attributable to the occupational environment and not to stimuli encountered outside the workplace. In addition, pre-existing asthma may be provoked by exposure at work. Occupational asthma may occur immediately or after a latent period of months or years in the same occupation. A very large number of agents may act as provocative agents for occupational asthma. The agents which are recognised for compensation in the UK are shown in **Fig. 6.12**.

Higher molecular weight compounds act through specific IgE and there may be long latent periods, over 10 years in some cases, before asthma develops. Lower molecular weight compounds act as haptens and require proteins for antibody formation. Other low molecular weight compounds such as diisocyanates follow an allergic clinical pattern, but the precise mechanisms are unknown. Other substances such as formaldehyde can act as direct irritants through non-immunological mechanisms.

Detection of occupational asthma depends on a careful history and the monitoring of PEF, both at work and away from exposure. Once an occupational sensitivity has developed there will usually be increased sensitivity to other non-specific and allergic triggers of asthma. Peak flow rates should be recorded regularly, up to every two hours. Monitoring should be continued during weekends, but it may require a longer period away from work to demonstrate the pattern clearly (**Fig. 6.13**).

Isolation of the specific cause of occupational asthma may require identification of specific antibody through skin or blood tests or challenge with suspected agents in the laboratory. Such challenges should be done carefully since they can produce severe or delayed reactions.

Agents provoking occupational asthma, officially recognised for compensation in UK
• Isocyanates
• Soldering flux (colophony)
• Stainless steel welding
• Platinum salts
• Epoxy resin hardening agents
• Azodicarbonamide (PVC, plastics)
• Glutaraldehyde
• Persulphate salts
• Reactive dyes
• Proteolytic enzymes
• Drug manufacture (antibiotics, cimetidine, ispaghula, ipecacuanha)
• Animals/insects used as laboratory animals
• Animals/insects, larval forms
• Crustaceans
• Flour/grain dusts
• Castor bean dust
• Wood dust
• Soya bean dust
• Tea dust
• Green coffee beans

Fig. 6.12. Agents provoking occupational asthma which are officially recognised for compensation in the UK.

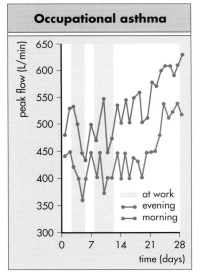

Fig. 6.13. Occupational asthma. PEF monitoring in a patient who worked as a paint sprayer. The shaded area represents his periods at work, and his PEF fell over these periods. It improved at the weekend amd, more markedly, during a two-week vacation. The patient was allergic to isocyanate, used as an activator in spray paint.

Numerous agents which are not on the prescribed list have been related to occupational asthma. Control of industrial processes and the environment reduce exposure and prevent the onset of problems, as does appropriate protective apparatus in some occupations (**Fig. 16.18**). In addition dusty, cold or polluted environments at work may exacerbate asthma through non-specific means.

INFECTIONS

Most patients report that an upper respiratory infection leads to an exacerbation of their asthma. Some of the symptoms of such an infection, including sneezing, cough and rhinorrhoea, may also be produced by exposure to an allergen. Studies of infections which exacerbate asthma show that the responsible organisms are usually viruses, particularly rhinoviruses, influenza, parainfluenza and respiratory syncitial virus. Airway reactivity may increase after a viral infection (**Fig. 6.14**).

EXERCISE

Formal exercise testing will provoke a drop in PEF in over 80% of childhood asthmatics. Two main theories of the mechanism exist, both based around the hyperventilation of exercise. One theory invokes heat loss from the airway mucosa as the main cause, the other water loss producing hypertonicity in the mucosa. Exercise-induced asthma is prevented by breathing warm, moist air and is exacerbated by exercise on a cold dry day. Swimming in a warm indoor pool is least likely to produce exercise-induced asthma.

Unlike many other challenges to the airway, exercise does not sensitise the airway to other triggers and does not result in a late response. Asthmatics should be encouraged to exercise normally after taking adequate preventative medication. A warm up period reduces the effects of subsequent exercise.

CLIMATE

Cold air is able to provoke asthma even without exercise. Thunderstorms have been associated with increased presentations with acute asthma (*see* **Fig. 6.8**). One reason may be that rapid humidity changes result in the rupture of pollen grains and mould spores, which pressure changes have trapped at low levels in the atmosphere.

POLLUTION

Much attention has been paid to the effects of pollution in recent years (**Fig. 6.15**). A number of studies have shown that various forms of pollution can increase the symptoms of asthma. Higher levels of ozone can sensitise the airway to other triggers; sulphur dioxide, oxides of nitrogen and particulates have all been linked

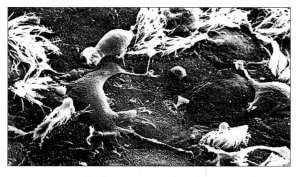

Fig. 6.14. A viral infection may induce damage and expose the underlying nerve endings. This illustration shows a bovine trachea after viral infection. The epithelial cells are shed exposing the submucosa and the nerve endings, which explains the increased airway reactivity after such infections. This usually returns to normal in 6–10 weeks.

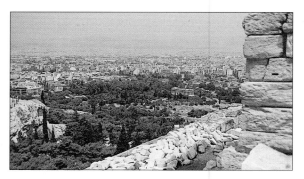

Fig. 6.15. A number of components of air pollution have been related to exacerbation of asthma. Oxides of nitrogen and sulphur dioxide levels have been related to symptoms and drops in peak flow rate. High levels of ozone are associated with increased problems with asthma a day or so later. Levels of small particulate matter have been related to cardio-respiratory deaths. Some cities such as Athens have very high pollution levels because of their climate, geographical situation and high traffic load.

to increases in respiratory symptoms, and there is a relation between particulate levels and deaths from cardiorespiratory disease. Indoor pollution from cooking fuels has also been associated with asthma problems. The place of pollution as an inducer, and thus in changes in the prevalence of asthma, is still unclear, however (*see* page 12).

SMOKING

Some studies have shown that 15–20% of asthmatics continue to smoke, although this delivers a far greater level of pollution to the lungs than any provided in the environment. Patients with asthma should not smoke. Passive smoking has been associated with worsening of asthma and parental smoking may increase the prevalence and the severity of asthma in children, so the homes of asthmatics should be smoke-free.

EMOTION

Emotional factors are unlikely to produce asthma on their own, but can interact with other causes to exacerbate the condition. Asthma may be provoked by actions such as laughing or crying, but this may result from the sudden intake of cold air. Social and psychological factors are very important in the management of asthma. They are relevant to compliance with treatment, and poor asthma control and even asthma deaths have been linked to psycho-social problems.

SLEEP

There is a diurnal rhythm of airway calibre in asthma. This is an amplification of a slight change seen in normal subjects, and the diurnal variation in PEF can be used in the diagnosis of asthma, and as a guide to the adequacy of control. Diurnal variation in the activity of the sympathetic and parasympathetic systems and in the inflammatory changes in the airways may all be involved.

HORMONAL CHANGES

The control of asthma often changes during pregnancy. It may either improve or worsen and subsequent pregnancies may not share the same pattern. Changes in asthma control may also occur at the menopause and with menstruation. Some women find that appreciation of their asthma symptoms changes with the menstrual cycle, without an associated change in PEF.

THYROTOXICOSIS

Severity of asthma may change with thyroid status, worsening with thyrotoxicosis and improving if the thyroid is underactive. This will not influence the thyroid treatment, but may help to explain changes in asthma control.

GASTRO-OESOPHAGEAL REFLUX

Gastro-oesophageal reflux of acid can exacerbate asthma (**Figs 6.16, 6.17**). This may occur through aspiration or laryngeal stimulation. There is also some evidence that receptors in the oesophagus itself can induce cough and airway narrowing in response to acid reflux.

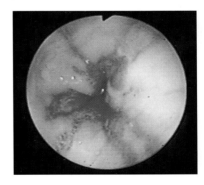

Figs 6.16, 6.17. **Gastro-oesophageal reflux** may provoke asthma symptoms. Reflux causes symptoms as acid leaves the stomach. **Fig. 6.16** shows linear ulceration of the oesophagus. **Fig. 6.17** shows simultaneous pH recordings with probes at 5 cm above the lower oesophageal sphincter (upper trace) and 2 cm above the upper oesophageal sphincter (lower trace). This shows that the patient has gastro-oesophageal reflux and also gastro-oesophago-pharyngeal reflux, which is particularly likely to cause bronchoconstriction and cough.

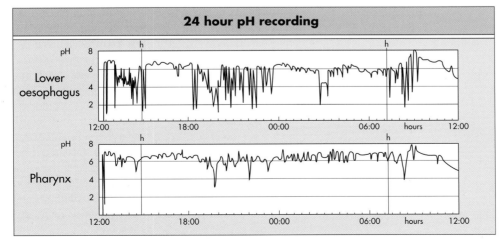

7 INVESTIGATIONS

RESPIRATORY FUNCTION TESTS

The most important investigations in a patient with newly diagnosed asthma are the history and the assessment of the degree of obstruction from peak flow or other respiratory function measurement (**Fig. 7.1**, *see* Chapter 4). Continued monitoring of PEF, often including home monitoring (*see* page 73), and of the results of other respiratory function tests is also of great importance in the long-term management of asthma (*see* page 102).

A number of other investigations may also be useful at the time of diagnosis, during acute exacerbations, or for monitoring the course of asthma.

Common tests of respiratory function

Test	Abbreviation	Result in asthma
Peak expiratory flow	PEF	Reduced in proportion to obstruction
Forced expiratory flow in one second	FEV$_1$	Reduced in proportion to obstruction
Forced vital capacity	FVC	Reduced in moderate, severe asthma
Relaxed vital capacity	RVC	Equal to FVC
Total lung capacity	TLC	Mild increase in moderate, severe asthma
Residual volume	RV	May increase if > mild asthma
Functional residual capacity	FRC	May increase if > mild asthma
Maximum expiratory flow at lower lung volumes	MEF$_{50}$, etc.	Reduced early in asthma
Airways resistance	Raw	Increased
Specific conductance	sGaw	Increased
Transfer factor	TLCO	Normal or reduced in proportion to reduction in volume
Transfer factor per unit lung volume (diffusion coefficient)	KCO	Normal or increased

Fig. 7.1. **Common tests of respiratory function.** The most useful tests in asthma are repeated measurements of PEF and FEV$_1$. Other tests are useful in differentiating asthma from other causes of dyspnoea.

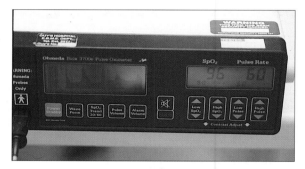

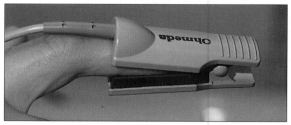

Fig. 7.2. **Pulse oximeter.** The widespread introduction of pulse oximeters has been a great benefit in many areas of medicine. The estimation of oxygen saturation is not accurate at very low levels, but the areas of interest in asthma are over 80% saturation. In this range the common oximeters are accurate if cardiac output and local circulation are adequate.

OXYGEN

Measurement of blood gases is important in the assessment of acute asthma when hypoxia and hypocapnia are usual findings. Hypercapnia is a danger sign that the attack is very severe and that exhaustion may be setting in. If the arterial carbon dioxide level is not raised initially then the oxygen saturation can be followed by pulse oximetry as long as there is no clinical deterioration (**Fig. 7.2**). In stable asthma estimation of blood gases is not necessary. In patients with a substantial irreversible element oximetry is useful, but this should be supplemented by estimation of blood gases if the saturation when breathing room air is less than 93%. A prior record of normal blood gases in patients with severe or 'brittle' asthma may aid the interpretation of results when the patient has an acute exacerbation.

BLOOD EOSINOPHILS

The blood eosinophil count is often raised in asthma (**Fig. 7.3**). Very high counts are not usually seen in asthma unless there are complications such as allergic broncho-pulmonary aspergillosis (ABPA, *see* page 32) or the asthma is part of another condition such as Churg–Strauss syndrome (*see* page 48). Tropical worm infestations such as *Ascaris* may be associated with eosinophilia and urticaria. Treatment of asthma with steroids usually produces a prompt reduction in the blood eosinophil count.

SPUTUM

The yellow or green colour of infected sputum is produced by degenerating white cells. The sputum in asthma may be yellow or green even in the absence of infection, since the same colours may be produced by the presence of high numbers of eosinophils in the sputum (**Fig. 7.4**). Microscopy of sputum is not a routine investigation in asthma, but sputum production can be induced in most patients by the inhalation of nebulised hypertonic saline, and research is in progress into the possibility that the examination of cell counts (**Fig. 7.5**), immunohistochemistry and mediator levels in such 'induced' sputum could provide a non-invasive method to follow the course of airway inflammation in asthma.

LUNG BIOPSY AND BRONCHOALVEOLAR LAVAGE

These techniques are not used routinely in asthma, but they are important in basic research into mechanisms and the effects of therapy. Biopsies may be studied by light microscopy, electron microscopy (*see* **Figs 2.3, 2.8**) or immunohistochemistry (*see* **Fig. 3.7**). Bronchoalveolar lavage (BAL) involves the washing out of a portion of the airways via a bronchoscope. Cell counts (**Fig. 7.5**), immunohistochemistry and mediator levels can be measured in the BAL fluid, and their course with time or their response to therapy can be followed.

RADIOLOGY

The chest radiograph in asthma is often normal. In acute exacerbations hyperinflation may be obvious with descent of the right diaphragm below the anterior end of the sixth rib. The posterior ribs may appear horizontal with the increased lung volume. In chronic uncontrolled asthma in children there may be permanent effects on the rib cage, but such changes are rare (**Fig. 14.11**).

Mucus plugging of airways may produce areas of linear atelectasis or localised infiltration. More prominent changes may be seen with the plugs of ABPA (*see* page 32).

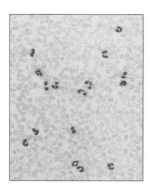

Fig. 7.3. Blood eosinophilia is a common finding in asthma. Very high levels are found in Churg–Strauss syndrome (allergic granulomatosis).

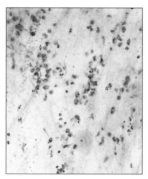

Fig. 7.4. Sputum eosinophilia is common in asthma. Large numbers of degenerating eosinophils produce a yellow or green colour in the sputum which mimics infected sputum. Eosinophilic sputum may contain crystalline structures, Charcot Leyden crystals, which are composed of the protein products of degranulated eosinophils.

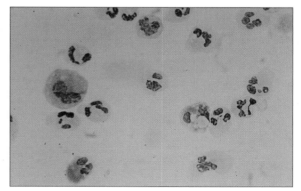

Fig. 7.5. Inflammatory cells in a sample of induced sputum from a patient with asthma. Sputum may be induced by the administration of nebulised hypertonic saline in 80% of normal individuals and almost all asthmatics. Centrifugation of the suspended cells ('cytospin') allows their microscopic and histochemical examination. This sample shows a macrophage and a number of polymorphs (mainly neutrophils). The mediator content of the supernatant can also be examined. Similar techniques can be used on samples obtained by the more unpleasant technique of bronchoalveolar lavage (BAL).

One of the anxieties in acute asthma is that a pneumothorax may be missed (**Fig. 7.6**). With an overinflated resonant chest with quiet breath sounds the clinical signs of a pneumothorax may be difficult to detect. Pneumothorax and pneumomediastinum are rare complications of acute asthma, and a chest radiograph can be deferred until the initial management is under way unless there is a strong suspicion of pneumothorax. Chest radiographs in the acute attack may show areas of segmental collapse secondary to plugs of sputum, and rarely this can produce collapse of a whole lobe or lung through a plug in a central bronchus (**Figs 7.7, 7.8**).

Radiology may be necessary to explore other areas such as the spine in chronic severe asthma, when vertebral collapse or osteoporosis induced by long-term oral steroid therapy is suspected (*see* **Fig. 16.27**).

SKIN TESTS

Many asthmatic patients are atopic: they have a tendency to make IgE in response to common inhaled allergens. This can be investigated by skin prick tests, in which a tiny quantity of allergen is introduced into the superficial layers of the stratum corneum (**Fig. 7.9**).

A true positive skin prick test reaction (**Figs 7.10, 7.11**) indicates that specific IgE is fixed to mast cells in the skin and has led to a vasoactive response due to release of histamine. When the allergen concentration is high, or the patient's sensitivity is extreme, a late skin reaction may also follow 4–6 hours (or even as late as 24–48 hours) after the test, with erythema, swelling and induration. This may be particularly significant in the investigation of ABPA (*see* page 32).

When carefully performed, using good preparations in the correct concentration, with appropriate positive

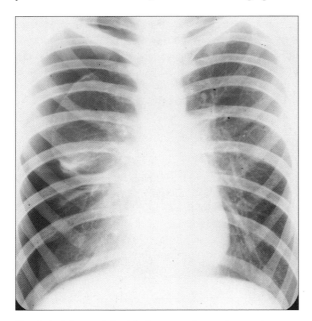

Fig. 7.6. A large right-sided pneumothorax in a patient with asthma. Spontaneous pneumothorax and pneumomediastinum are rare complications of acute attacks of asthma

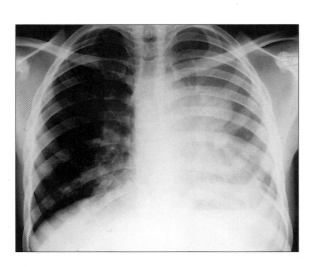

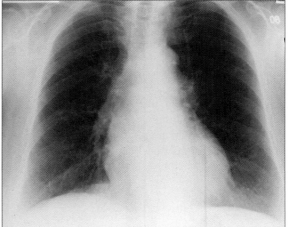

Figs 7.7, 7.8. Left upper lobe collapse and recovery associated with bronchial plugging. Chest radiographs in an adolescent with poorly controlled asthma. He noticed increased breathlessness and vague left-sided chest pain before the first radiograph was taken (Fig. 7.7, left). Later he coughed up a firm rubbery lump of material, the symptoms improved and the left upper lobe re-expanded (Fig. 7.8, right).

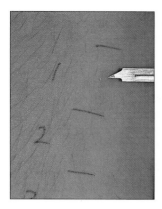

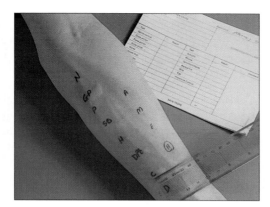

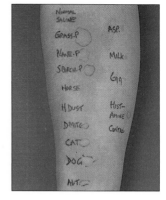

Fig. 7.9. Skin prick testing is useful in asthma. The volar surface of the forearm is cleaned, prick sites are marked, and drops of the relevant allergen extracts in appropriate concentration are placed on the skin. The test should always include a negative control of 0.5% phenol saline, the suspending solution for the allergens, and histamine 1% as a positive control. A lance or a standard needle is introduced through each drop at 45° to the skin surface to a depth of about 1 mm, the skin is lifted slightly, and the lance withdrawn. The procedure is painless, and the puncture sites should not bleed. The skin is blotted dry, and the resultant reaction is assessed at 15–20 minutes (*see* **Fig. 7.10**).

Fig. 7.10. Reading the skin prick test results. The maximum reaction is usually seen after 15–20 minutes. The saline control (N) should be negative (unless the patient has dermographism—*see* **Fig. 7.13**). The histamine control (H) should be positive—recent antihistamine administration may cause a negative result, and this invalidates other negative reactions. The presence of a positive skin response indicates the presence of specific IgE antibody in the blood, and there is a reasonable correlation between the size of the weal and the significance of different inhaled allergens in a single patient. Positive results are best recorded by measuring the diameter of the weal in millimetres, using a transparent gauge or a ruler. Here the strongest reaction is to grass pollen (GP), and significant positive reactions are also seen to cat (C) and the house dust mite *Dermatophagoides pteronyssinus* (Dpt). The interpretation of the response depends on the clinical history.

Fig. 7.11. Multiple positive skin test results. Many asthmatics have multiple positive skin test reactions to common allergens, showing the ease with which they make IgE antibodies to common allergens in the environment. This British patient had positive reactions to grass, plane and silver birch pollens, cats, dogs and *Alternaria*. All may contribute to his asthma, which is perennial with a tendency to seasonal exacerbations during the period from April to August. The other allergens gave negative results—the flare reactions should be regarded as non-specific (a common reaction in patients with eczema), and there was no measurable weal.

(histamine) and negative (diluent) controls, skin test results correlate well with the results of bronchial challenge testing (which cannot be performed routinely), and thus give useful information on the allergens involved in asthma; but the results must always be correlated with clinical history. For inhaled allergens, up to 15% of positive results are false positives, but fewer than 5% of negative results are false negatives. However, skin testing is relatively unreliable for ingested allergens including food, partly because of the nature of the available allergen preparations and partly because reactions to ingested substances are not always mediated by IgE.

Only a small number of allergens are needed for routine skin prick testing in patients with asthma. A typical skin test battery can include four antigens, together with positive and negative controls (**Fig. 7.10**). Additional antigens can be added when there

is a clear possibility of the involvement of other antigens (**Fig. 7.12**). It is important to remember that a number of less common allergens may also cause asthma. These include cockroaches (in inner-city areas in the USA), soya bean dust (responsible for epidemics in Barcelona), fungi (including *Didymella, Alternaria* and even *Trichophyton* – the cause of athlete's foot), latex, hair-care products and peanuts. The role of some of these allergens cannot be successfully investigated by skin prick testing; occupational allergens are also usually better identified by other means (*see* **Fig. 6.13**).

Although it is wise to perform skin tests in a medical setting in which adrenaline and basic resuscitation skills are available, the risk of systemic reaction from skin testing with the usual antigens is extremely low. They are, however, contra-indicated in the presence of

Allergen extracts commonly used in skin testing
Routine short screen for atopy:
Phenol saline (negative control) Histamine (positive control) House dust mite* Grass pollen** *Aspergillus fumigatus* Cat
Additional allergens which may be used:
Tree/weed/other plant pollens *Alternaria* *Cladosporium* Dog Any other relevant animals Any relevant foods Any other relevant inhaled allergens
* Mixed 'house dust' extracts may be used in the routine screen; alternatively specific allergens from *Dermatophagoides pteronyssinus* and/or *Dermatophagoides farinae* may be used. ** In some regions it is appropriate to include an alternative pollen antigen in the routine screen (e.g. birch in Scandinavia, ragweed in North America). The mix of grass pollens used may also vary between regions.

Fig. 7.12. Allergen extracts commonly used in skin testing.

widespread eczema, in which false-positive results and exacerbation of eczema are common sequels; and they are of no value in patients with dermographism (**Fig. 7.13**).

Skin tests can be economically and widely used, and they provide information which is valuable in the management of most patients with asthma (**Fig. 7.14**).

Skin test results in an individual patient do not usually change radically, but they tend to become less marked with age, and new positive responses may appear if there is some new exposure from the environment. Skin tests do not usually need to be repeated unless a new allergen is suspected.

IgE MEASUREMENTS

Total IgE levels are commonly raised in asthma and it is also possible to look for specific IgE by radio-allergo-sorbent testing (RAST). A high level of total IgE can be a cause of false-positive specific RAST results. Like skin prick tests, the RAST shows the presence of specific IgE, but does not necessarily indicate that the particular allergen is an important cause of the patient's asthma. In the investigation of occupational asthma there may be many more workers with specific IgE than with demonstrable asthma. The sensitivity and the specificity of the RAST depends upon the quality of the allergen used. The interpretation of the result depends upon the clinical situation.

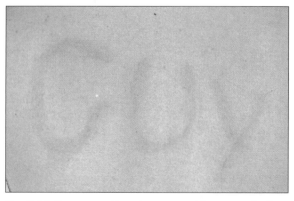

Fig. 7.13. **Dermographism** demonstrated by writing firmly with a finger on the back of a patient at a well-known London teaching hospital. Patients who produce a prominent weal in response to minor stimuli may give positive skin test responses to the trauma of the needle prick in skin testing. However, dermatographism should be suggested by a positive response to the diluent used as the negative control.

The value of skin prick tests in the management of asthma
• Positve tests are diagnostic of atopy, and suggestive of the provoking and perpetuating cause(s) of asthma. • Uniformly negative tests exclude allergens as a significant factor in most patients with asthma. • Skin tests provide supportive evidence (positive or negative) for the clinical history. • Skin tests provide valuable corroboration of allergy before embarking on difficult or expensive avoidance measures, e.g. for house dust mites. • Skin tests have useful educational and confirmatory value for the patient, providing a visual reinforcement of verbal information and advice.

Fig. 7.14. The value of skin prick tests in the management of asthma.

8 DIFFERENTIAL DIAGNOSIS

CHRONIC OBSTRUCTIVE PULMONARY DISEASE

Chronic obstructive pulmonary disease (COPD) consists of a combination of chronic bronchitis and emphysema. Chronic bronchitis is characterised by chronic or recurrent cough with excess sputum production in the absence of any other cause (**Fig. 8.1**). The epidemiological definition of chronic bronchitis requires sputum production for 3 months of 2 consecutive years.

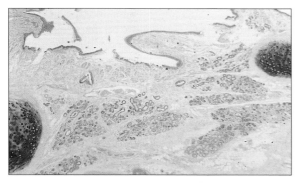

Fig. 8.1. A large airway in chronic bronchitis. In COPD hyperplasia of the mucus glands in the airway wall results in excess mucus production. Abnormal ciliary action, sticky mucus and patchy cilial loss all impair muco-ciliary clearance.

Emphysema has a pathological definition based on enlargement of air spaces distal to the terminal bronchiole, with destruction of the alveolar walls (**Figs 8.2, 8.3**). The two conditions can occur in isolation but usually co-exist in varying proportions in COPD. Tobacco smoke is the main cause of COPD, but other factors such as pollution or hereditary deficiencies of α-1-antitrypsin are responsible in some cases. Around 20% of smokers have an accelerated decline of lung function which will end in symptomatic COPD if they continue to smoke. It is not known why the majority of smokers are not susceptible to COPD, although they retain the risks of cardiovascular disease and of lung and other cancers from their smoking.

Cough and sputum develop early and are more common than airway obstruction in COPD. The faster decline of FEV_1 in the susceptible subset of smokers produces the first signs of breathlessness at the age of 40–50 years. Eventually this may go on to respiratory failure and cor pulmonale.

COPD may be difficult to differentiate from chronic asthma in adults. On occasions asthma may go unrecognised by patient and doctor and even present with right heart failure secondary to chronic hypoxia and pulmonary hypertension. The main features which help to

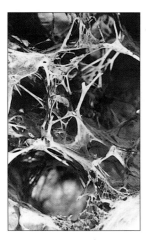

Fig. 8.2. Severe emphysema in a lung section. In milder disease the changes may be localised to a centra-acinar distribution or be periacinar. In severe emphysema no pattern is recognisable. There are large bullae with residual fibrous bands. Lack of lung support and alveolar structure lead to expiratory airflow obstruction and reduced gas transfer.

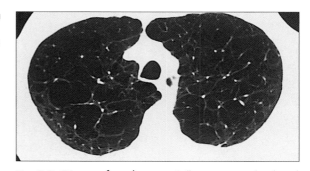

Fig. 8.3. CT scan of emphysema. Bullous areas and reduced density of the lung structure are well shown on thin slices of lung in a CT scan. This has emerged as the best method for quantification of the extent of emphysema. The measurements of density correlate well with histological findings.

differentiate the conditions are the history of smoking, which is usual in COPD, and the degree of reversibility with bronchodilators and steroids in asthma. The borderline between asthma and COPD is debatable, and it is not clear whether a reversible element to airway obstruction can occur in pure COPD or always implies co-existent asthma. The so-called 'Dutch hypothesis' suggests that it is the smokers who start with increased bronchial reactivity who are susceptible to the effects of tobacco smoke.

The main purpose of a differentiation between asthma and COPD is to ensure that appropriate treatment is given. Asthmatics with persistent symptoms should receive regular inhaled steroids. There is no firm evidence that this is also appropriate for COPD, but some studies have suggested this, and several large international trials are addressing this point. If these studies show that regular anti-inflammatory treatment is appropriate in COPD then the differentiation from asthma will become more blurred and less important. Meanwhile it is important to explore the reversibility of all patients with airway obstruction and the effects of a trial of inhaled steroid when the obstruction is persistent. This pragmatic approach should achieve all

possible reversibility but leaves the issue of regular long-term inhaled steroids unresolved.

CYSTIC FIBROSIS

Cystic fibrosis is the commonest severe recessively inherited condition amongst Caucasians, with a prevalence rate of 1 in 2000. While most patients present in childhood with typical problems of malabsorption, intestinal obstruction and repeated chest infections, a minority present in their teens or twenties (**Figs 8.4, 8.5**). Chest symptoms tend to predominate in these milder cases and cough and wheezing may be the main symptoms. Wheezing is also a common symptom in infants, positive skin tests are common and 20% of cystic fibrosis patients are reported to have co-existent asthma.

Cystic fibrosis can be detected by an abnormally high sweat sodium. In adolescents and adults this test is less reliable, but it may be improved by prior treatment with fludrocortisone. Alternatively, the measurement of transepithelial potential difference in the nose is available in special centres and a value above 35 mV is both sensitive and specific for cystic fibrosis.

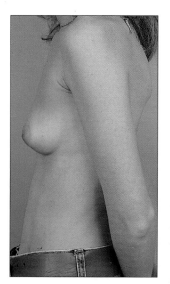

Fig. 8.4. Cystic fibrosis. Wheezing and positive skin tests can occur in cystic fibrosis and a sweat test should be performed if this diagnosis is suspected. In older patients and in milder cases the sweat test may not be diagnostic. If the level of suspicion is high then the common cystic fibrosis genetic abnormalities should be sought or the nasal potential difference can be measured in specialised centres. This 18-year-old girl had intercostal recession and signs of weight loss (loose trousers and belt). In mild cases and in some older children and adults bowel symptoms may be absent and nutrition may not be a problem.

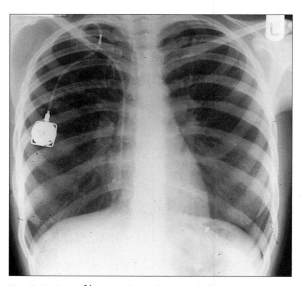

Fig. 8.5. Cystic fibrosis. The radiological changes usually start in the upper lobes with ring and tubular shadows from thickened bronchial walls and more confluent shadows from obstructed airways. This girl has an indwelling intravenous line, Portacath, for administration of antibiotics at home.

LARGE AIRWAY PROBLEMS

Obstruction of a large airway can mimic asthma and such conditions are often treated with bronchodilators for weeks or months before the correct diagnosis is made. Large airway obstruction occurs with tumours of the larynx, trachea or main bronchi or with benign lesions. The trachea may be narrowed after endotracheal intubation or tracheostomy. Crico-arytenoid disease in rheumatoid arthritis can narrow the larynx. Arteritic conditions such as Wegener's granulomatosis or relapsing polychondritis can affect the airways at any level. Occasionally endobronchial tuberculosis or sarcoidosis produce large airway problems.

Clues to the site of the obstruction are an inspiratory wheeze, stridor or a typical appearance on the flow–volume loop (**Figs 8.6–8.8**) or even on a spirometry trace (**Fig. 8.9**).

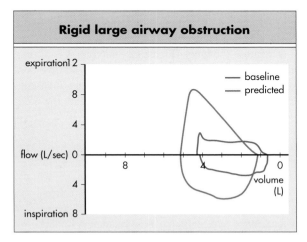

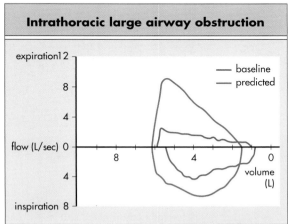

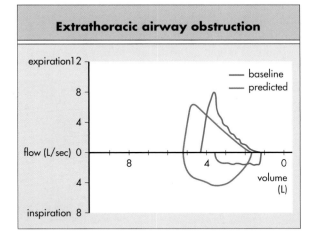

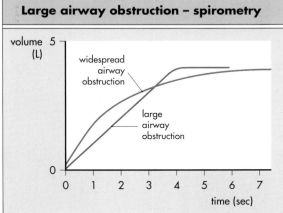

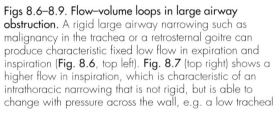

Figs 8.6–8.9. Flow–volume loops in large airway obstruction. A rigid large airway narrowing such as malignancy in the trachea or a retrosternal goitre can produce characteristic fixed low flow in expiration and inspiration (**Fig. 8.6**, top left). **Fig. 8.7** (top right) shows a higher flow in inspiration, which is characteristic of an intrathoracic narrowing that is not rigid, but is able to change with pressure across the wall, e.g. a low tracheal stricture after prolonged intubation. In **Fig. 8.8** (bottom left) the expiratory flow is fixed but the inspiratory flow is higher suggesting an extrathoracic lesion such as a laryngeal narrowing. The volume–time trace from a spirometer in a case of large airway obstruction is shown in **Fig. 8.9** (bottom right) with that of an asthmatic for comparison. A straight line on the spirometer trace should always raise the suspicion of a large airway problem.

FOREIGN BODY

In children, aspiration of a foreign body can produce wheezing with no obvious history (**Figs 8.10, 8.11**). Wheezing may be localised to one lung and an expiration chest radiograph may help by showing that one lung does not deflate normally on expiration. Occasionally adults may aspirate a piece of bone and present days or weeks later with cough and wheeze but with little recollection of any earlier choking episode. The memory will be even hazier if the aspiration was associated with a high alcohol consumption.

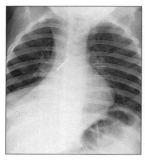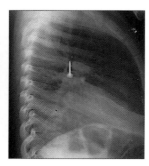

Fig. 8.10. A metallic foreign body aspirated in to the lungs will usually show on the chest radiograph. This nail is lodged in the right lower lobe bronchus.

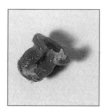

Fig. 8.11. A radiolucent inhaled foreign body. Objects such as this pen top aspirated by a child may produce shadowing in the obstructed segment or will need to be detected by clinical signs such as a localised wheeze or by failure to deflate on a radiograph taken in expiration.

ALLERGIC GRANULOMATOSIS

Allergic granulomatosis or Churg–Strauss syndrome occurs on a background of asthma which has usually been difficult to control and present for a year or more. A high blood eosinophilia is found, and tissue eosinophilia, granulomata and vasculitis develop in various organs. The lungs (**Fig. 8.12**), nervous system, skin and heart are often involved, while renal involvement is not usually significant (unlike other forms of vasculitis). Treatment is with systemic steroids, with the addition of azathioprine if necessary.

HEART FAILURE

Left heart failure causes shortness of breath from pulmonary oedema. This has been known as cardiac asthma since wheezing may be a prominent finding. The paroxysmal nocturnal dyspnoea associated with heart failure may be mistaken for the worsening of asthma in the early hours of the morning. Examination, chest radiograph (**Fig. 8.13**) and response to bronchodilators or diuretics should allow the two to be differentiated.

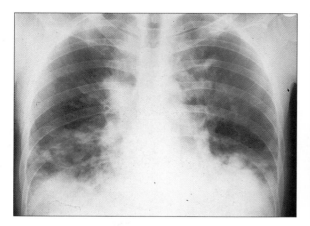

Fig. 8.12. Allergic granulomatosis (Churg–Strauss syndrome). Widespread lung infiltrates during a first episode of allergic granulomatosis. This was associated with poorly controlled asthma for one year, pericarditis and an eosinophilia of 12×10^9/L. Recurrences occurred when the dose of oral prednisolone was reduced below 15 mg daily.

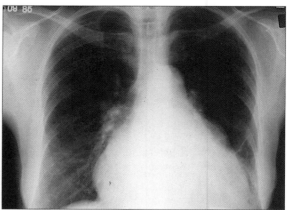

Fig. 8.13. 'Cardiac asthma'. Enlarged left atrium and ventricle in a woman with mixed mitral valve disease. The left atrial enlargement shows as a bulge on the left heart border from the left atrial appendage and a double shadow at the right heart border. Elevated pulmonary venous pressure and pulmonary oedema cause breathlessness and can produce prominent wheezing in some patients.

9 CLINICAL PHARMACOLOGY

INTRODUCTION

For most of the 20th century, asthma has been regarded as a condition in which symptoms and signs result from bronchospasm due to excessive contraction of the smooth muscle in the bronchial and bronchiolar walls. This belief formed the basis for the use of bronchodilator therapy with adrenergic agents, xanthine derivatives and anticholinergic agents, all of which commonly relieve the immediate symptoms of asthma.

The development of selective inhaled β_2-agonist agents, such as terbutaline and salbutamol, in the 1960s was a major advance in the symptomatic treatment of patients with asthma, and the regular use of such inhaled agents formed the 'core' treatment for most patients with mild to moderate asthma during the 1970s and 1980s.

Long-acting oral preparations of β_2-agonist drugs were also developed, though their use was often limited by systemic side effects; and, especially in North America, long-acting oral theophylline became another commonly used first-line therapy.

During the 1960s, 1970s and early 1980s, the predominant mechanism in asthma was commonly thought to be an interaction between inhaled allergen and surface mast cells. This was thought to lead to the release from mast cells of mediators, such as histamine, which caused bronchoconstriction.

Sodium cromoglycate was introduced in the early 1970s as an inhaled agent which is believed to inhibit the activation and release of mediators from mast cells, and it proved to have a preventive effect in some patients.

Antihistamine therapy was found to be ineffective in asthma, but this was potentially explicable by the involvement of other mediators released by mast cells, the effects of which were not blocked by antihistamine therapy. As discussed in Chapter 3, however, the theory that mast cells are largely responsible for the symptomatology of asthma has been severely challenged more recently as a result of the failure of a number of mast-cell stabilising compounds to have any significant clinical effect in asthma.

Despite the undoubted value of bronchodilator agents in the management of mild to moderate chronic asthma and acute severe asthma, it has always been clear that, even in the maximum tolerated doses, they are not fully effective in many patients. Where they are apparently effective, there is no evidence to suggest that they influence the natural history of the disease process. They often relieve the acute symptoms of asthma, but their continued use does not prevent future relapse, and some patients develop severe chronic symptoms, associated with a progressive decline in respiratory function, despite the continued administration of bronchodilator agents.

Since its development in the early 1950s, systemic steroid therapy has been an important and often life-saving therapy in patients with severe asthma. Its long-term use has, however, been limited by major unwanted effects. These severe side effects were the major stimulus to the development of inhaled steroid preparations, which have been widely used in patients with severe asthma since the 1970s. Many controlled clinical trials have established that inhaled steroids are effective in controlling asthma symptoms and in reducing the frequency of acute exacerbations.

Inhaled steroids represent the best available preventive treatment for most patients with asthma, and concern about side effects is probably largely unfounded when inhaled steroids are used in the normally recommended doses.

Drug therapy in asthma	
Preventive therapy	
Inhaled steroids	Oral methylxanthines*
Inhaled cromones	Oral leukotriene antagonists
Oral steroids	Oral steroid-sparing agents
Reliever therapy	
Inhaled β-agonists	Oral (or injected) β-agonists
Inhaled anticholinergics	Oral (or injected) methylxanthines
* Methylxanthines are viewed principally as reliever therapy, but may also exert a preventive, anti-inflammatory effect.	

Fig. 9.1. Drug therapy in asthma.

Nevertheless, future developments in drug therapy are likely. These may include the development of steroids which bind selectively to the respiratory mucosa and/or are metabolised locally or in the blood to inactive metabolites, and the development of other drugs which are active against mediators which are important in asthma, such as leukotriene antagonists.

At present it is important to consider the fundamental distinction between preventive (or prophylactic) therapy and reliever (symptomatic) therapy (**Fig. 9.1**).

PREVENTIVE THERAPY

Steroids

Glucocorticosteroids (steroids) were used in the treatment of chronic and acute asthma very soon after their development in the early 1950s. Dramatic improvements in the morbidity of many chronic asthmatics occurred, but were accompanied by systemic side effects. The use of the inhaled route did not initially reduce the systemic side effects because the steroids used were not metabolised by the liver; nor were they topically potent. The balance of wanted and unwanted effects changed dramatically with the introduction of topically potent inhaled steroids (e.g. beclomethasone dipropionate and budesonide), especially where high first-pass metabolism to inactive compounds has been demonstrated (e.g. budesonide and fluticasone).

Mechanism of action

Knowledge of the mechanism of action of steroids has increased over the past decade with the understanding of the role of transcription and translation of messenger RNA (mRNA) and synthesis of new proteins.

There is only one known type of glucocorticosteroid (GCS) receptor, and this is found in most cells in the body—which explains the widespread effects of systemic steroid therapy. Steroids are lipophilic, and they cross the cell membrane rapidly to enter the cytoplasm. Here, they combine with GCS receptors (**Fig. 9.2**). The protein molecules which have held the receptor in an inactive state (heat shock proteins) disassociate, and the GCS-receptor complex enters the cell nucleus.

In the nucleus the GCS-receptor complex acts as a transcription factor, binding to specific recognition sequences on the DNA in the promoter region of steroid-responsive genes. This interaction with DNA leads to target gene activation or suppression. Changes in gene transcription lead to an increase or decrease in specific mRNA production, and thus to an increase in the production of some anti-inflammatory mediators (and other proteins), and to a decrease in the production of pro-inflammatory mediators, including all known cytokines (**Fig. 9.2**). This decrease in cytokine production as a result of decreased transcription is probably an important action of steroid therapy in asthma, but other actions and interactions are also significant.

It is now clear that cytokines also act on cells by changing gene transcription. Their interaction with receptors on the cell surface leads to activation of the transcription factors NF-κB and activating protein (AP)-1. These then move to the nucleus and bind to DNA in the same way as the GCS-receptor, thus influencing mRNA production and influencing the production of proteins by the cell (**Fig. 9.3**).

The GCS-receptor can interact directly with both AP-1 and NF-κB in the nucleus (and even with the cytoplasm

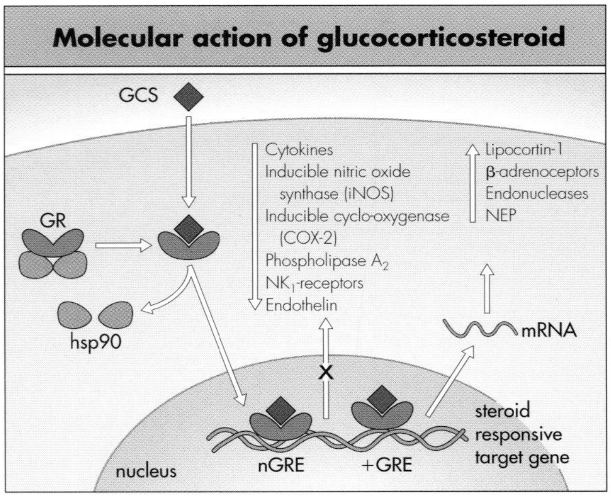

Molecular action of glucocorticosteroid

Fig. 9.2. The molecular mechanism of action of glucocorticosteroid (GCS). The GCS crosses the cell membrane to the cytoplasm, where it becomes bound to the GCS receptor (GR). The heat shock protein (hsp 90) molecules which have held the receptor in an inactive state dissociate from the GCS-receptor complex and the drug-receptor complex forms a dimer which crosses the nuclear membrane to act as a transcription factor, binding to the promoter-enhancer region of sensitive genes. This binding leads to a down-regulation of specific messenger RNA (mRNA) production, and thus to the down-regulation of the production and release of pro-inflammatory cytokines and other proteins. GCSs also lead to up-regulation of the production of a number of anti-inflammatory mediators, by increasing specific mRNA production for these mediators. (nGRE = negative glucocorticoid responsive element; +GRE = positive glucocorticoid responsive element.) (Adcock and Barnes, *Trends Pharmacol Sci* 1993;**14**:436–41).

Steroids and transcription factors

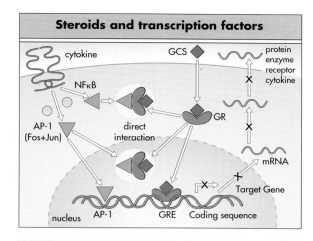

Fig. 9.3. Transcription factor–steroid receptor interaction. The interaction of cytokines with receptors on the cell surface leads to activation of the transcription factors NF-κB and activating protein (AP)-1. In the absence of exogenous steroid, these move to the nucleus and bind to DNA in the same way as the GCS-receptor complex, thus influencing mRNA production and the production of proteins by the cell. In the presence of exogenous steroid, the GCS-receptor complex can interact directly with both AP-1 and NF-κB in the nucleus (and with NF-κB in the cytoplasm), thus preventing their action as transcription factors, and effectively blocking the effects of cytokines on the cell. This protein–protein interaction is now believed to be one of the most important mechanisms in the anti-inflammatory action of steroids in asthma. (GRE = glucocorticoid responsive element.) (Adcock and Barnes, *Trends Pharmacol Sci* 1993; 14:436–41).

Key properties of the commonly used inhaled steroids				
Steroid	Water solubility (µg/ml)	Relative receptor affinity	Relative topical blanching potency in man[1]	Oral bioavailability
Beclomethasone dipropionate (BDP)/ Beclomethasone monopropionate (BMP)[2]	0.1/10	0.4/1.1[3]	0.6/0.4	–[4]
Budesonide	14	1[3]	1	6–13%
Fluticasone propionate	0.04	2.3[5]	1.2	~1%

[1] The blanching potency is a measure of anti-inflammatory effect.
[2] Beclomethasone dipropionate (BDP) is rapidly metabolised in the body to the active compound beclomethasone monopropionate (BMP).
[3] In human lung tissue.
[4] No published data.
[5] In rat thymus.

Fig. 9.4. Key properties of the commonly used inhaled steroids. (Data from Brattsand and Ingell, In: *Respiratory Allergy: Advances in Clinical Immunology and Pulmonary Medicine*, Eds Melillo, O'Byrne and Marone, Elsevier Science Publications, Amsterdam, pp. 129–36 and Bye, *Br J Clin Pharmacol* 1993;36:136–7.)

for NF-κB), thus preventing their action as transcription factors, and effectively blocking the effects of cytokines on the cell (**Fig. 9.3**). This protein–protein interaction is now believed to be a very important mechanism in the anti-inflammatory action of steroids in asthma. NF-κB and AP-1 mediate chronic inflammatory effects, and their inactivation 'switches off' the process.

Another major effect of steroids is to increase synthesis of β-receptors and restore down-regulated β-receptors seen in asthmatics receiving regular β-agonists.

Pharmacology of oral and topical steroids
The properties and potencies of commonly used inhaled steroids are shown in **Fig. 9.4**. The high topical potency for the inhaled steroids correlates with their local efficacy, and fluticasone and budesonide also have the advantage of high first-pass metabolism (**Fig. 9.5**). The swallowed portion (80–90% of the dose delivered by pMDI) is absorbed but mainly inactivated on first pass.

Systemic availability of an inhaled drug

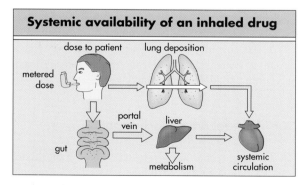

Fig. 9.5. The systemic availability of an inhaled drug is the sum of its absorption from the gastrointestinal and respiratory tracts. After absorption via the gut wall and liver, intact drug which escapes first-pass metabolism reaches the systemic circulation. Absorption via the lungs results in the direct entry of the drug into the systemic circulation. For inhaled steroids with very high first-pass metabolism (e.g. fluticasone, budesonide), this means that most systemic activity results from the portion of the dose deposited in the lungs.

With these inhaled steroids, the risk of unwanted systemic effects through gastrointestinal absorption is very small.

The preferred steroid for oral use is prednisolone, which can be given once a day because of its biological half life. If it is taken in the morning there is less suppression of the hypothalamic pituitary adrenal (HPA) axis. Short (< 3 weeks) courses of oral prednisolone are not associated with significant adrenal suppression. Long term oral steroid use has a wide range of side effects which include not only adrenal suppression, but Cushingoid facial features (**Fig. 16.25**), centripetal obesity, striae, skin atrophy (**Fig. 16.26**), hypertension, diabetes, osteoporosis (**Fig. 16.27**), and growth impairment in childhood (**Fig. 9.6**). Achilles tendon rupture, myopathy and altered body hair have all been reported.

Systemic side effects are much less common with inhaled steroids. They are rarely seen when normal therapeutic doses are used, but some systemic effects may be seen when inhaled steroids are used in high dose for prolonged periods of time. These side effects are substantially less than those which would be induced by the dose of oral steroids required to achieve the same degree of asthma control.

The risk of systemic side effects with inhaled steroids is influenced by several factors:
- The dose – higher doses are more likely to lead to systemic effects.
- The drug – different inhaled steroids may have different potential for systemic effects, related to their lipophilicity, tissue binding, first pass and systemic metabolism.
- The device used to deliver the drug. Increased lung deposition may lead to a greater risk of systemic effects if the dose is not correspondingly reduced.

Overall, in routine clinical practice, the risk of significant systemic side effects from inhaled steroids used in recommended doses is usually very low.

Non-steroidal prophylactic agents

The first non-steroidal prophylactic agent, other than antihistamines, to be introduced was the cromone sodium cromoglycate (SCG), which inhibits release of mediators from mast cells, as well as blocking activation of mast cells by other stimuli. Inhaled SCG may have an inhibitory effect on many inflammatory cells but its precise mechanism of action is unclear. SCG given before allergen challenge blocks the usual airway reaction, including the late asthmatic reaction, but SCG does not

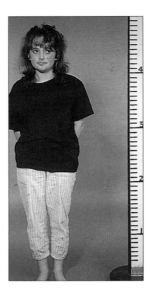

Fig. 9.6. Growth retardation in an 18-year-old girl with chronic asthma. This patient has failed to grow, is around 1.5 m (4 ft 10 inches) tall and has a 'high' hairstyle to give an impression of height. She received oral steroids throughout puberty, as inhaled topical steroids did not control her asthma. Severe asthma itself impairs growth, and it is often impossible to disentangle the relative effects of oral steroids and asthma on growth. Inhaled steroids in normal doses have been shown not to impair linear growth in childhood (see Chapter 15).

block the effect of histamine challenge. It also blocks exercise-induced asthma. The four-times-a-day regimen required for maximum efficacy is difficult to follow, but apart from local irritation and cough, the drug seems free from the risk of serious side effects.

Nedocromil sodium, another cromone, is a pyrenoquinolone dicarboxylic acid which has been shown to have a large number of effects on inflammatory cells and models of asthma, in particular inhibition of histamine, leukotriene C_4 and prostaglandin D_2. Nedocromil sodium has similar blocking action to sodium cromoglycate but appears to be more potent. Both sodium cromoglycate and nedocromil sodium may have an additional inhibitory effect on sensory nerve fibres in the lung. Airway responsiveness to metacholine is significantly reduced after 8 weeks of treatment with nedocromil. Although nedocromil has a significant therapeutic effect in atopic and non-atopic asthmatics, there is a lack of comparative studies with other anti-inflammatory agents. Like SCG, it has a good safety profile, with only a bad taste and occasional local irritation as side effects.

Ketotifen is a potent H_1-antagonist and is often effective in rhinitis and urticaria. Although it blocks acute allergen and histamine challenge, its overall clinical efficacy in asthma is weak. The studies which show greatest benefit suggest that clinical efficacy takes at least 2 months of treatment. Sedation occurs in 10–20% of patients, particularly adults, and there may be associated weight gain as ketotifen is an appetite stimulant.

Leukotriene antagonist and 5-lipoxygenase inhibitors

Recently, drugs active on the 5-lipoxygenase pathway have been developed. Some, such as zafirlukast, inhibit the action of leukotrienes LTD_4 and LTE_4 at the receptor, while zileuton is an inhibitor of the 5-lipoxygenase enzyme. Challenge studies looking at the effect of exercise, cold air and allergen-induced asthma have suggested some efficacy. However, not all asthma is leukotriene mediated; in exercise-induced asthma and cold air-induced asthma, the most potent LTD_4 receptor antagonists leave residual bronchoconstriction. Zafirlukast and other LTD_4 antagonists have a small but significant effect on bronchoconstriction which is less (under half) that of β-agonists, but this 'bronchodilator' effect is additive to that of β-agonists. There are few long-term studies using leukotriene antagonists in chronic asthma so their role in day-to-day management of asthma is unclear, but apparent safety and early suggestions of efficacy suggest that they may have a role in the future.

Immunosuppressive agents

Several immunosuppressive agents have been used in patients with severe asthma, in the hope of reducing or eliminating the need for systemic steroid therapy.

Methotrexate

Methotrexate is a dihydrofolate reductase inhibitor, decreasing folate production and thus preventing biosynthesis of thymidylate and purines which leads to decreased synthesis of DNA and RNA. As a consequence, T-lymphocyte replication and function, basophil histamine release, neutrophil chemotaxis and interleukins (IL) will be inhibited. Although usually used in high doses for cancer chemotherapy, in low dose (15–30 mg weekly) methotrexate has been proposed for severe asthma. Side effects, particularly impairment of liver function, pulmonary fibrosis and *Pneumocystis* pneumonia, suggest that there are no clear indications for methotrexate in asthma.

Cyclosporin

Cyclosporin A is a cyclic peptide from a fungus that appears to prevent the activation of T lymphocytes. Clinical trials give conflicting evidence of its efficacy and further trials are awaited before its role in asthma is clarified. Side effects, particularly on renal function and blood pressure, and the need to monitor cyclosporin levels, prevent its regular use.

Other drugs

Gold, azathioprine and troleandomycin have all been suggested as additional immunosuppressive agents but their side effects, monitoring requirements and little data suggesting efficacy mean they have no current role in the management of asthma.

RELIEVER THERAPY

β-Agonists

Selective $β_2$-agonists are the mainstay bronchodilator agents for the treatment of asthma, in very mild asthma, in acute exacerbations and in the prevention of nocturnal asthma (long-acting $β_2$-agonists).

Adrenoreceptors were originally divided into α– and β-receptors, but β-receptors were subsequently divided into $β_1$ and $β_2$. More recent studies have suggested a metabolic $β_3$ effect. Smooth muscle within the airways contains almost exclusively $β_2$-receptors while in terminal airways there are both $β_1$- and $β_2$-receptors. Epithelial and mucosal glands and mast cells also have $β_2$-receptors so $β_2$ drugs may also affect mucus secretion and mediator release from mast cells.

β-Agonist binding to the β-adrenoreceptor requires activation of an intermediary protein before stimulating adenylcyclase leading to production of cyclic AMP (cAMP). The cAMP leads to activation of protein kinase A with the range of cellular effects shown in **Fig. 9.7**. β-Receptors can exist in high or low affinity states, the former having 5–100 times the affinity for agonists. Prolonged exposure to high concentrations may lead to down-regulation, although steroids and the large spare receptor capacity may preserve the tissue response such as the bronchodilatation to a given dose.

β-Agonists consist of a benzene ring with a chain of two carbon atoms and either an amine head or a substituted amine head (**Fig. 9.8**). When hydroxyl (-OH) groups are present in positions 3 and 4 on the benzene ring the compound is termed a catecholamine and has high potency. Repositioning of these hydroxyl groups (e.g. in salbutamol and terbutaline) reduces potency but also reduces metabolic degradation by catechol-O-methyltransferase (COMT) and allows increased length of action compared with isoprenaline.

Effects of β-receptor activation

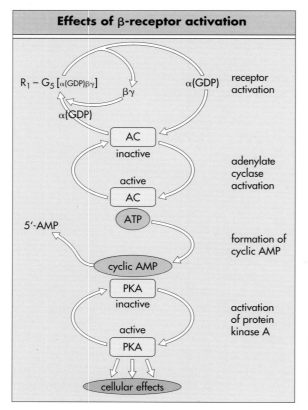

Fig. 9.7. Schematic representation of effects of β-adrenoceptor activation. Following binding of agonist, the receptor–G$_s$ complex releases GDP allowing GTP to bind resulting in the dissociation of the α subunit of G$_s$, which is responsible for activating adenylate cyclase (AC). AC catalyses the conversion of ATP to cyclic AMP, which in turn activates protein kinase A (PKA) leaing to the intracellular effects of cyclic AMP. Following activation of AC, the α subunit of G$_s$ recombines with GDP and the βγ subunits producing the inactive form of G$_s$. Cyclic AMP is broken down by non-selective and cyclic AMP-selective phosphodiesterases to 5'-AMP.

Structure of some β-agonists

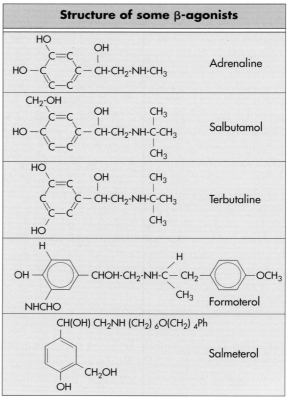

Fig. 9.8. Structure of some β-agonists.

Alterations in the amine head increase β$_2$-selectivity and affect resistance to activation by monoamine oxidase which, like COMT, is widely distributed in the lung.

Long-acting β-agonists

Formoterol and salmeterol have a prolonged length of action but the mechanism for this is unclear, although both drugs are more lipophilic than short-acting agents and are therefore likely to have a more non-specific cell membrane binding. Salmeterol has a large polar N substituent and may interact with non-polar groups on the receptor protein. The length of action of formoterol is only sustained via the inhaled route and may be due to the addition of a pyridine nucleus. The long-acting oral drug bambuterol is a pro-drug of terbutaline. As a result of slow absorption, a combination of oxidative and hydrolytic metabolism, and a reversible selective inhibitory action on plasma cholinesterase, bambuterol acts as an 'inner depot' from which terbutaline is gradually generated.

Duration of action may also be lengthened by increasing the dose. For example, 5 mg of salbutamol has a considerably longer action than 0.2 mg, the usual inhaled dose from a pMDI.

Side effects

β-Agonists cause a wide range of metabolic changes but the only clinically significant effect is the fall in serum potassium. A fall in serum potassium of 0.4–0.9 mmol/L occurs with single doses from lowest inhaled dose to the highest intravenous dose. Fine tremor can be a nuisance with oral or high dose inhaled β-agonists (**Fig. 9.9**), although it tends to decrease with prolonged treatment as tolerance develops.

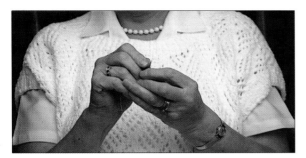

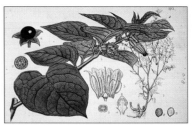

Fig. 9.10. *Datura stramonium* (belladonna, deadly nightshade). A natural source of the anticholinergic drug atropine.

Fig. 9.9. Short-term and long-term side effects of β-agonists are increasingly recognised. There are many metabolic side effects but in most situations these are not clinically significant, apart from fall in serum potassium. Muscle tremor, however, can affect fine hand movement activities, as in this patient who is a seamstress and finds threading needles and fine sewing difficult. Tolerance may develop but is not necessarily total.

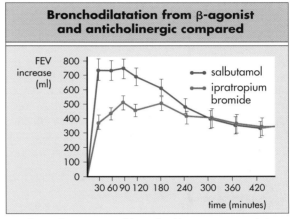

Bronchodilatation from β-agonist and anticholinergic compared

Fig. 9.11. Comparison of bronchodilatation rate and size of response to salbutamol and ipratropium bromide. (Modified from Thiessen and Pedersen, *Respiration* 1982; **43**:304–16.)

Safety of β-agonists

β-Agonists given by inhalation have a very high short-term safety profile but there are concerns about long-term safety. Temporal relations with asthma deaths in the 1960s and again in the late 1970s with isoprenaline and fenoterol respectively have been noted, but proving a causal relationship has been more difficult. There are a number of potential mechanisms; the most obvious is the failure to take other treatments, particularly prophylactic anti-inflammatory or oral steroids during an exacerbation.

Tolerance has been shown with rebound bronchial hyperresponsiveness following withdrawal of the β-agonist. The effects appear small, but may be significant in a small minority. Evidence that β-agonists cause significant dysrhythmias is conflicting, although angina, ST elevation on ECG and clinically non-significant cardiac arrhythmias have been demonstrated with high dose β-agonists and with lower doses in conjunction with methylxanthines. Recently, the racemic nature of many β-agonists has been investigated, with one isomer considered as a bronchoconstrictor while the other isomer is the more potent bronchodilator. If tolerance develops to the latter, bronchoconstriction may be dominant.

Anticholinergics

Anticholinergic compounds such as the herb *Datura stramonium* (**Fig. 9.10**) and belladonna powder were used as inhaled or oral preparations early in the 19th century. The introduction of the safer adrenoreceptor stimulants led to reduced use until the development of quaternary ammonium derivatives of atropine such as ipratropium bromide and oxitropium bromide with their far greater safety.

Anticholinergic (antimuscarinic) drugs antagonise the effects of acetylcholine at muscarinic cholinergic receptors. Subtypes of muscarinic receptors have been recognised, with the subtypes M1, M2 and M3 found most commonly in the lung. M3 is the major subtype which leads to airway muscle contraction. Both M1 and M3 are associated with increased secretion of mucus. Ipratropium bromide and oxitropium bromide act as non-selective blockers. They have reduced lipid solubility and therefore do not cross the blood–brain barrier easily. The minimal proportion (5%) systemically absorbed is metabolised while the majority of the drug is excreted in the faeces.

Bronchodilatation starts early after inhalation of either of these two compounds, but does not reach maximal effect until 45–90 minutes (**Fig. 9.11**) and lasts 4–6 hours for ipratropium bromide and longer for oxitropium bromide. Mucociliary clearance is not affected by these drugs, unlike atropine.

Side effects at low dose are mainly limited to a dry mouth or unpleasant taste but occasional cases of paradoxical bronchoconstriction have been reported. High doses, particularly via a nebuliser, should be given with caution in patients with glaucoma, prostatic hypertrophy or a history of cardiac arrhythmias. Combination therapy with β-agonists produces an additive effect.

Methylxanthines

The best known methylxanthines are three naturally occurring substances found in food and beverages: theophylline, caffeine and theobromine. Although caffeine is recognised to have bronchodilating properties, theophylline has been used for the treatment of asthma and remains the most widely prescribed anti-asthma treatment worldwide. Theophylline, although an effective bronchodilator, is less potent than β-agonists, and with the introduction of inhaled steroids its use has declined in many countries.

Mechanism of action

Despite their long history, the molecular mechanisms responsible for the therapeutic effect of methylxanthines remain unclear. Phosphodiesterase (PDE) inhibition has been suggested as the means for bronchodilator activity, but the degree of inhibition is small at therapeutically relevant concentrations of theophylline. Isoenzymes of phosphodiesterase have been identified: PDE III is predominant in airways smooth muscle and PDE IV on mast cells, eosinophils and T lymphocytes. Although theophylline is non-selective, there is some evidence that PDE isoenzymes may have an increased expression in asthmatics. This is supported by the lack of bronchodilator effect in normals, compared with that in asthmatics.

Adenosine-receptor antagonism, increased catecholamine release and inhibition of calcium ion flux have all been proposed as mechanisms of action for theophylline. More recently, effects of theophylline on inflammatory cells *in vivo* have been identified at concentrations lower than those usually considered necessary for bronchodilation (5–10 mg/L compared to 12–20 mg/L). Potentially helpful effects on reducing inflammatory mediators have been noted on mast cells, neutrophils, monocytes, macrophages, eosinophils and T lymphocytes (**Fig. 9.12**). T lymphocytes may orchestrate the eosinophilic inflammation found in asthma and this immunomodulatory mechanism may explain some of the efficacy of theophylline on asthma symptoms in patients on low doses.

Pharmacokinetics, physiological and drug interactions and side effects

Methylxanthines are irritant when inhaled and are used orally or intravenously, the latter in acute severe asthma. The therapeutic range has been based on the degree of active bronchodilator following administration. This range of 12–20 μg/L is associated in a significant proportion of patients with side effects, particularly nausea, headache and central stimulation with insomnia. In the UK, theophylline has been prescribed primarily as a bronchodilator, following the introduction of slow-release formulations to maintain steady but high serum concentrations. These formulations reduced the swinging levels of the previous tablet and suspension preparations but may have lost favour because of the high incidence of side effects. Even at the lower concentrations being suggested for the immunomodulatory action there is significant variability in absorption, with both physiological and drug interactions. Side effects such as convulsions and cardiac arrhythmias may occur because drug interactions can often lead to high serum concentrations. Careful prescribing and knowledge of factors leading to reduced metabolism are important, but with its comparatively low cost and the increase in asthma worldwide, the immunomodulatory action of theophylline deserves further research.

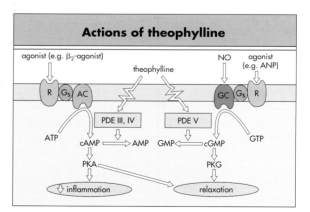

Fig. 9.12. Action of theophylline as a phosphodiesterase (PDE) inhibitor. PDE III and PDE IV break down cyclic adenosine-3′,5′-monophosphate (cAMP), whereas PDE V breaks down cyclic guanosine-3′,5′-monophosphate (cGMP). Theophylline is a nonselective PDE inhibitor and therefore increases cAMP and cGMP levels, resulting in bronchodilation and inhibition of inflammatory cells. AC: adenylate cyclase; ATP: adenosine triphosphate; GTP: guanosine triphosphate; R: receptor; GC: guanyl cyclase; G$_s$: stimulatory G-protein; PKA: protein kinase A; PKG: protein kinase G; ANP: atrial natriuretic peptide.

10 DRUG DELIVERY IN ASTHMA

Drugs may be administered to the asthmatic patient by three main routes: orally, by injection and by inhalation.

Oral and injected therapy are usually administered in the same way to patients with asthma as to those with other disorders, so they are covered briefly here. The principles of inhaled therapy are, however, of fundamental importance to the management of most patients with asthma, so they are discussed in more detail.

ORAL THERAPY

Many believe that the ideal therapy for asthma – as for other chronic disorders – would be a once-daily oral preparation. The quest for such effective, safe and simple therapy is still in progress, but has not yet been fulfilled. The reliever drugs used in asthma have short half-lives, and many different slow-release preparations of methylxanthines and β-agonists have been developed over the past 20 years. The aim is to maintain constant drug levels throughout the day without toxic peaks and sub-therapeutic troughs.

There are two main types of slow-release preparations: wax-like matrices, in which the drug leaches out slowly over a period of time; and osmotic pump capsules where the drug is continuously released through a small hole (**Fig. 10.1**).

Steroid therapy may, of course, be given orally, but its use is restricted to acute severe asthma and to patients with intractable disease, because of the inevitability of side-effects with long-term treatment (**Figs 9.6, 16.25–16.27**).

For routine management of asthma inhaled therapy is generally preferable to oral treatment with the advantages of low, targeted dose, reduced side effects and, in the case of the β-agonists as rescue medication, speed of onset.

INJECTED THERAPY

Aminophylline, β-agonists and steroids may all be given by injection in acute severe asthma (*see* Chapter 17), but the use of injected therapy is rarely necessary in other situations.

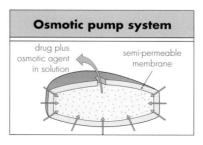

Fig. 10.1. Osmotic pump system. A capsule for the delivery of oral salbutamol, using an osmotic pump to produce sustained release of the drug.

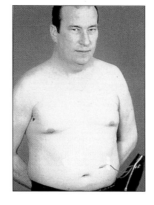

Fig. 10.2. A patient with severe 'brittle' asthma receiving continuous subcutaneous β₂-agonist via a small battery-driven syringe pump. A very few patients may be dramatically helped by continuous subcutaneous selective β₂-agonist beta stimulant. This patient varied the dose in a similar fashion to a diabetic between day and night and his morning PEF dips were stopped.

Self-administered subcutaneous or intravenous β-agonists have been used successfully in afew patients with brittle asthma. Fears of downregulation of β-agonist receptors remain, but in occasional patients chronic administration via continuous subcutaneous infusion is the only effective treatment (**Fig. 10.2**). The high doses used lead to muscle tremor and, in some patients, agitation. Subcutaneous nodules may develop at the injection site.

In some patients with severe life-threatening asthma attacks who, as a result of repeated use of intravenous lines, have poor venous access, the insertion of a Hickman line or Portacath indwelling catheter may be life-saving (**Fig. 10.3**).

INHALED THERAPY

Local treatment of the respiratory tract with drug aerosols has a history which stretches back for at least

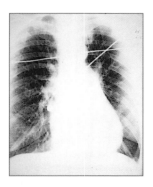

Fig. 10.3. A chest radiograph showing the insertion of intravenous line which has a diaphragm below the skin. The patient's peripheral veins have been destroyed by the multiple previous hospital admissions and the severity of her asthma is such that without immediate venous access for therapy she has severe life-threatening attacks.

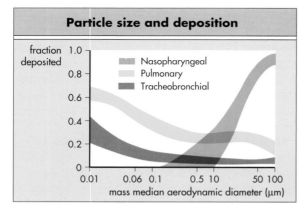

Fig. 10.4. Inhaler devices in asthma. This picture includes just some of the many devices available, including various pMDIs, spacer devices, dry powder inhalers and nebuliser chambers. Note the inclusion of an metal spacer device to the right. The drug delivery and clinical performance of these inhalers varies widely and in many cases has not been fully assessed.

100 years, but its major role in the management of asthma and other respiratory disorders has only developed over the past 40 years. The introduction of the pressurised metered-dose inhaler (pMDI) in 1956 allowed effective portable aerosol administration for the first time; and the development of progressively more specific and effective anti-asthma therapy and of new forms of inhalers during the 1970s and 1980s led to many potential improvements in quality of life for the typical patient with asthma. The wide range of inhalers now available may, however, cause confusion for prescribers and patients (**Fig 10.4**).

Pressurised metered-dose inhaler (pMDI)

For inhaled therapy to be effective, the drug must be able to reach the airways (**Fig. 10.5**), and this requires a particle diameter < 5 µm (**Fig. 10.6**). Larger particles than this are mainly deposited in the upper airway and then swallowed. The optimal site of deposition is assumed to be the small airways and it is not known whether deposited drug is locally transported to other airway sites.

To generate the correct particle size and deliver this to the airway, most pMDIs contain the drug substance, up to three propellants and one or two surfactants and lubricants. These ensure aerosolisation of the drug on release and also lubricate the valve mechanism. The valve mechanism (**Fig. 10.7**) allows the release of the aerosol in individual aliquots. Most anti-asthma drugs are available in

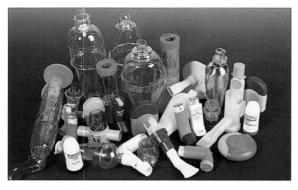

Fig. 10.5. The effect of particle size on deposition within the respiratory tract. Deposition in the respiratory tract can be predicted from the International Committee on Radiation Protection model for three compartments. Such models and radio-labelling techniques show that aerosol sizes of a mass median diameter of 3–5 µm are the most suitable for bronchodilator aerosols.

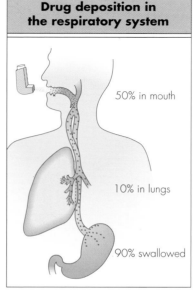

Fig. 10.6. Drug deposition in the respiratory tract after using a metered dose aerosol. Only 10% of the drug from a pMDI reaches the lung, 50% is impacted within the mouth and, due to the larger particle size being deposited in the oropharynx and not inhaled, overall 90% of the drug is swallowed.

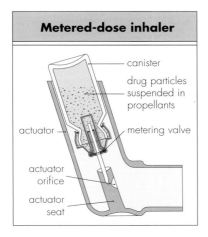

Metered-dose inhaler

- canister
- drug particles suspended in propellants
- actuator
- metering valve
- actuator orifice
- actuator seat

Fig. 10.7. Pressurised metered-dose inhaler (pMDI). A metered dose of drug is released on pressing down the canister against a spring loaded valve. The active drug is mixed with propellant(s) and surface active agent(s) to prevent aggregation of the drug.

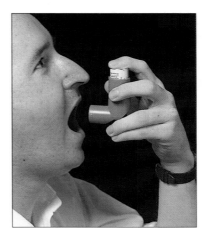

Fig. 10.8. pMDI using HFA 134A. A pMDI using HFA 134A as the propellant. The appearance and mode of use of the new pMDIs is similar to those propelled by CFCs, but their performance characteristics may be different.

pMDI forms and with appropriate care and the correct technique pMDIs are effective. However, there are two important disadvantages:

- Even after strenuous efforts at education, some patients are unable to co-ordinate inhalation with actuation of the pMDI.
- The usual propellants in pMDIs are chlorofluorocarbons (CFCs).

CFCs are being phased out because of their damaging effect on the ozone layer in the stratosphere. Alternative propellants are the hydrofluoroalkanes HFA 134A and HFA-227 (also known as hydrofluorocarbons; HFCs). New pMDIs using these propellants are becoming available (**Fig. 10.8**), but, although HFAs do not affect the ozone layer, they are recognised 'greenhouse gases' and may have an impact on global warming. Their use might also be curbed in the future.

There are several other significant problems with pMDI use:

- The patient may stop inhalation when the aerosol cloud hits the back of the throat (the 'cold freon' effect).

- Initial bronchoconstriction may occur, even when the drug is a bronchodilator.
- The delivered dose may vary, particularly when the pMDI is not properly shaken (**Fig 10.9**).
- It is difficult to assess how much drug content remains in the pMDI.

There is also concern over the dose variation between different manufacturers' pMDIs. The first dose released is often much lower in drug content than the second or third dose, even when the pMDI is correctly shaken. The cause of the variation is not fully explained but probably results from variations in design of the metering chambers. Drug delivery, particle size and lung deposition may be different in pMDIs utilising HFA propellants.

The problem of co-ordination in pMDI use may be overcome either by inspiratory firing of the pMDI, where the inhaled inspiratory flow triggers a spring mechanism which automatically fires the device releasing the aerosol (breath-actuated inhaler – **Fig. 10.10**), or by the addition of a large volume spacer device with an inspiratory/expiratory valve to the pMDI.

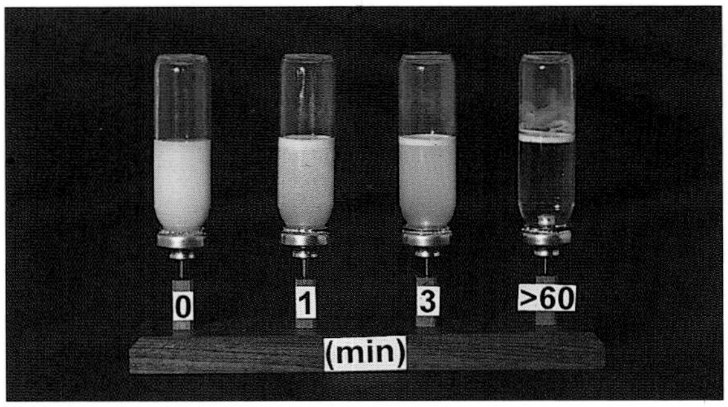

Fig. 10.9. Behaviour of the contents of a pMDI as revealed by using glass walled containers. This pMDI contains a suspension of micronised budesonide as used in production pMDIs. The pMDI was shaken at time 0 and the progressive separation of the contents over the ensuing hour is obvious, with complete separation after 60 minutes. Similar separation occurs in pMDIs containing most drugs, though some may sink rather than float.

Pressurised metered-dose inhalers with spacer devices

Large volume valved spacer devices (**Figs 10.4, 10.11, 15.9, 15.10, 16.22**) were originally introduced to allow the patient to breathe in the aerosol without the associated need to co-ordinate actuation of the pMDI with inhalation. The patient can actuate the pMDI once and then breathe tidally through the spacer, with a low resistance one-way valve preventing dilution of the drug and allowing maximal inhalation. A number of other advantages of spacer devices have now been recognised, although their size and relative lack of portability are a major disadvantage when they are used for relief therapy with short-acting bronchodilators. They are particularly useful in infants (**Fig. 15.9**).

Pressurised MDIs have a high initial velocity and the droplets have an initial mass median diameter (MMD) which is high (30 μm, well above the 'inspirable' particle size of 5 μm). These larger particles are deposited in the mouth and upper airway when a pMDI is used without a spacer device, leading to a risk of local side effects (a problem with inhaled steroids in particular) and reduced airway efficacy. As the velocity of the aerosol decreases within a spacer, the MMD also decreases (**Fig. 10.12**), the large particles either being deposited within the spacer or reduced in size by evaporation to a MMD < 5 μm and inspired.

The greater lung deposition and lower oropharyngeal deposition with large volume spacers is associated with a decreased risk of local and systemic side-effects and an increase in drug efficacy when compared with administration by pMDI without a spacer. Unfortunately, however, it is now clear that the dose received through a spacer is potentially widely variable. Polycarbonate spacers are initially highly electrostatically charged. Much of the first 10–20 doses of aerosol fired into a new spacer is deposited on its walls, as a result of this charge. As the spacer becomes well used, a greater proportion of each dose reaches the patient. At this stage, however, the spacer may be washed for hygiene reasons; washing and drying may restore the charge so that the cycle is repeated.

Multiple actuations into a spacer before inhalation may also lead to a relative decline in the delivered dose.

The use of new materials, such as metal (**Fig 10.4**), in the construction of spacers may overcome the problem of charging, but at present the clinical significance of 'dirty' versus 'clean' spacers is probably variable and difficult to assess.

Inspiratory flow driven dry powder inhalers

Inspiratory flow driven dry powder inhalers (DPIs) use the patient's inspiratory force to generate the drug aerosol.

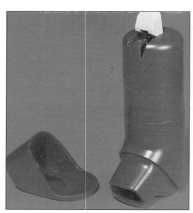

Fig. 10.10. Breath-actuated device. Breath-actuated devices are triggered by the start of inspiration by the patient and are actuated by such low inspiratory flow rates that they can be used as rescue bronchodilators as well as assisting in drug delivery to the lung in poor pMDI inspiratory co-ordination. The device here is open for use and the lever primed.

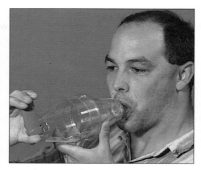

Fig. 10.11. Large volume 'spacer' or extension chamber added to metered-dose aerosol. Large volume spacers have a one-way respiratory valve which overcomes co-ordination problems, particularly in children. They may also be used in acute attacks of asthma to deliver repeat aerosol doses of bronchodilator every few minutes. Such spacer devices may also increase lung deposition and reduce oral impaction, a potentially useful feature with high-dose inhaled steroid therapy.

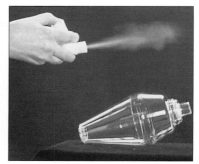

Fig. 10.12. Velocity and particle size following discharge from a pMDI. An aerosol plume following discharge from a pMDI demonstrating the reduction in velocity and droplet/particle size as the propellant evaporates and the aerosol reaches the level of the valve in the spacer device.

A number of difference types of DPI are now available. The original DPIs, including Spinhaler® (**Figs 10.13, 15.11**), Inhalator® and Rotahaler® (**Fig. 15.11**) require the individual loading of each dose in capsule form. More recent inhalers include a rotating capsule inhaler for ipratropium bromide (**Fig. 10.14**) and Diskhaler®, which is loaded with a disk of capsules containing 4–8 doses of drug (**Figs 10.15, 10.16, 15.11**).

Turbuhaler® (known as Turbohaler® in some countries) was the first truly multidose inhaler, and is preloaded with a reservoir containing up to 200 doses of drug (**Figs 10.15, 10.17, 10.18, 15.12**). The recently introduced Diskus® (also known as Accuhaler®) is another form of multidose inhaler (**Figs 10.15, 10.19**). Unlike Turbuhaler, it does not contain a single large reservoir of drug but multiple separately blistered doses which are released individually.

All these inhalers are breath actuated and require the patient to breathe in as quickly and deeply as is comfortable through the mouthpiece after the device has been loaded.

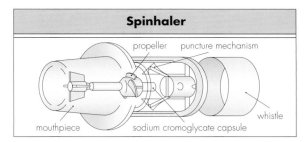

Spinhaler

propeller   puncture mechanism

mouthpiece   sodium cromoglycate capsule   whistle

Figs. 10.13. The original inspiratory flow driven dry powder inhaler (Spinhaler), used for the delivery of sodium cromoglycate. Each dose is loaded individually. The capsule is then pierced by a puncture mechanism and the powder inhaled by deep inspiration. Dispersion is achieved by a rotating spindle. Inspiratory flows must achieve a minimum rate. The addition of a device which generates a 'whistling' noise allows the patient and doctor to check that the inspiratory technique is adequate.

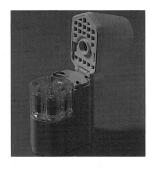

Fig. 10.14. Rotating capsule inhaler: A novel rotating capsule device for inhaling ipratropium bromide. The device holds six doses.

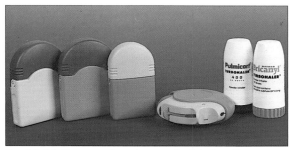

Fig. 10.15. Some modern dry powder inhalers. Two examples of the 8-dose Diskhaler (left), a 4-dose Diskhaler (centre), a Diskus (Accuhaler) and two examples of the Turbuhaler (Turbohaler). Diskus and Turbuhaler are true multidose inhalers.

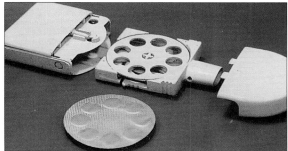

Fig. 10.16. Diskhaler: dry powder disk system. The Diskhaler can deliver 4–8 individual doses of drug (beclomethasone dipropionate, fluticasone, salbutamol, salmeterol) which are in blisters on a disk loaded into the inhaler. The disks are pierced and the drug (combined with lactose, a carrying agent) is inhaled. The disk is rotated to load the next dose when the device is closed, avoiding the need to load individual capsules.

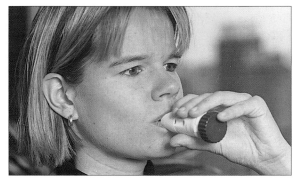

Fig. 10.17. Turbuhaler (Turbohaler): A dry powder, multi-dose inhaler. This inhaler is easy to use and high patient preference rates have been reported when compared to the pMDI. Turbuhaler can be used to deliver budesonide, terbutaline, salbutamol and – potentially – other drugs. When 20 doses remain a warning red marker appears, so a replacement may be obtained before the drug runs out.

Turbuhaler

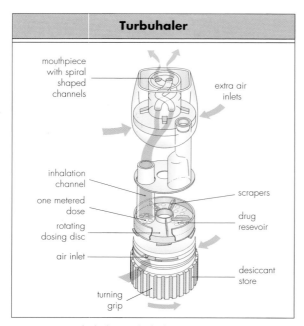

Diskus

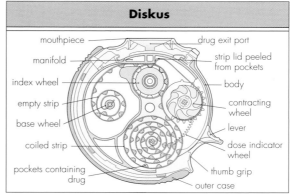

Fig. 10.19. Diskus (or Accuhaler). A new multidose dry powder inhaler, in which the dose of drug is sealed between two strips of material at regular intervals, and this roll is fitted inside. On actuation the two strips of material are separated releasing free drug to the mouthpiece where it can be inhaled. A dose counter shows the precise number of doses remaining in the inhaler.

Fig. 10.18. Turbuhaler (Turbohaler). The dose-metering mechanism in this inspiratory flow-driven multidose inhaler dispenses small quantities of drug to a high degree of accuracy. Turbuhaler is pre-loaded with up to 200 doses of budesonide, terbutaline or other drugs. Each dose is loaded by the patient before use by twisting the grip at the bottom with Turbuhaler held vertically, or at least 45° from horizontal. This process turns the dosing disk, which is situated below the drug reservoir, and the conical holes in the disk are filled with dry-powder compound from the reservoir. Scrapers remove excess drug from the disk. Inhalation draws air through Turbuhaler, carrying a metered dose of drug up through the mouthpiece and into the patient's airways. The spiral design of the mouthpiece creates turbulent airflow which breaks the drug into mainly small, respirable particles.

Rotahaler, Diskhaler and Diskus devices deliver a mixture of drug with a carrier powder, usually lactose. Carriers prevent aggregation of the drug but include large particles that are deposited in the upper respiratory tract and large airways; rarely, they may cause adverse effects like cough or bronchoconstriction.

Turbuhaler can deliver budesonide and terbutaline as pure drug substance, but a small amount of lactose may be necessary for the delivery of very small doses of drugs through this system.

Dry powder devices require a balance between inspiratory flow rates, built in resistance and the generation of some turbulent airflow so that there is maximum deaggregation of the dry powder at an inspiratory force that can be achieved by patients with asthma. Turbuhaler has a relatively high resistance to airflow because of the

spiral channels in the mouthpiece which are designed to generate turbulent flow and deaggregate the micronised drug. Rotahaler and Diskhaler have lower resistances but require relatively high inspiratory flow rates to generate an effective aerosol. In practice, most patients over the age of 4 or 5 can be trained to use most DPIs effectively, even during acute exacerbations of asthma.

Drug delivery to the lung from inhalers

With the proliferation of new delivery systems and the varying potencies of drugs, particularly steroids, it is important to be aware that not all drug delivery systems are the same, particularly in terms of the nominal dose leaving the inhaler device and that reaching the target organ. *In vitro* attempts to identify the likely proportion of drug reaching the lung can be assessed by impaction of the aerosol using a multistage Andersen sampler. Particles with a diameter of around 5 μm or less are most likely to be deposited within the lung.

In vitro, different pMDIs do not necessarily give similar fine particle doses of different drugs; different DPIs may produce different particle sizes (**Fig. 10.20**) and the drug delivered from different inhalers may thus have markedly different deposition patterns.

Deposition from different inhalers can also be assessed *in vivo* using scintigraphy, where the aerosol is prelabelled with particles containing a radio-isotope which emits γ-rays (these particles are in the same size range as the drug, but are not usually the drug itself).

The proportion of radiolabelled aerosol deposited at the various sites (inhaler, oropharynx, central and peripheral airways) may be assessed as shown in **Fig. 10.21**.

A less direct technique to estimate pulmonary deposition is to measure the systemically available drug after preventing absorption from the gastrointestinal tract by using activated charcoal given by mouth before the study. There are some differences between techniques but it is clear that the lung deposition from different devices and with different drugs varies widely. This has an effect on both the clinical response and the possibility of side effects. Dose adjustment may be possible or necessary when a patient switches from one inhaler to another, even if the prescribed drug is unchanged.

Delivery device, efficacy and side effects

When equal nominal doses of drug are administered, Diskhaler and Rotahaler produce about 50% of the lung deposition achieved by pMDI, whereas the addition of a large volume spacer device leads to greater lung deposition than with pMDI alone. By comparison, Turbuhaler administration results in a greater lung deposition than administration by pMDI.

For ß-agonist and anticholinergic inhaled drugs, the desired bronchodilator effect and any unwanted systematic effects are both closely related to the lung deposition of the drug.

The relationship between clinical efficacy, local side effects and systemic side effects is more complex with inhaled steroids. Beclomethasone dipropionate (BDP) is believed to have the lowest first-pass metabolism, so in doses over 1,000 µg/day may be associated with systemic side effects due to oropharyngeal deposition and ingestion of the drug. Mouth rinsing immediately after dosing may help to reduce these risks, but using a large volume spacer will have equal or greater effect by allowing the deposition of the larger aerosol particles in the chamber.

The first-pass metabolism of budesonide and fluticasone is very high, and the risk of systemic effects from these drugs results mainly from the lung-deposited fraction rather than the oropharyngeal component. The efficacy of budesonide administered via Turbuhaler often allows the dose to be halved, reducing the risk from systemic side effects.

Choosing the right inhaler is a complex task, requiring a balance between ease of co-ordination, the risk of local and systemic side effects, clinical efficacy and high compliance (**Fig. 10.22**).

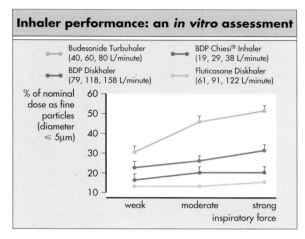

Fig. 10.20. Inhaler performance: an *in vitro* assessment. The proportion of the nominal dose as fine particles obtained in an Andersen sampler with four different dry-powder inhalers at flow rates corresponding to weak, moderate and strong inspiratory forces. The bars represent the standard deviation for the results from three inhalers of each type. (Olsson, *J Aerosol Med*, 1995; **8(Suppl 3):** S13–18.)

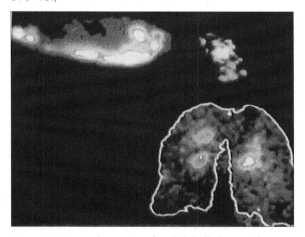

Fig. 10.21. Lung deposition of radiolabelled aerosol using a large volume spacer and pMDI. There is considerable deposition in the spacer, relatively low oropharyngeal deposition, and up to 30% of the delivered drug is deposited below the larynx with wide dispersal throughout the smaller airways.

Nebulisers

The use of nebulised therapy in the treatment of asthma has increased dramatically over the last decade. There are many reasons for this including the ability of nebulisers to deliver high doses of drug, particularly bronchodilators, comparatively quickly and to allow patients to receive treatment who are otherwise unable to inhale drugs (especially infants).

Two main types of nebuliser are available, jet and ultrasonic. The jet nebuliser, which is effective for all medications, including particulate suspensions such as inhaled topical steroids, is the most commonly used (**Fig. 10.23**). The larger droplets generated fall into the reservoir, the smaller droplets move with the gas flow to be inhaled. The multiplicity of jet nebulisers means that they have widely differing characteristics particularly with regard to the generation of droplets of a suitable particle size which can be inhaled into the lung.

The performance of nebulisers can be affected by a number of factors other than just the type of nebuliser used. The residual volume of the nebuliser is 0.5–1.5 ml. Although this may be reduced by tapping the nebuliser towards the end of nebulisation, adequate volume of fill is required to ensure drug delivery to the lung. The duration of nebulisation and the nature of the solution or suspension also affect nebuliser performance. However, the most important factor is the driving gas flow rate at which the nebuliser functions most efficiently. The nebuliser should be matched to the portable air compressor (**Figs 10.24, 15.7, 15.8, 16.24**). Portable mechanical air compressor systems are also available.

Ultrasonic nebulisers use high frequency sound waves produced from a piezoelectric crystal, which bounces on the surface of the liquid to generate a polydispersed aerosol. The aerosol size varies with the ultrasonic frequency but ultrasonic nebulisers tend to be less efficient than modern jet nebulisers, and they cannot be used to nebulise particulate suspensions.

Some advantages and disadvantages of the three forms of portable inhaler	
Advantages	**Disadvantages**
pMDI	
• Quick to use • Compact and portable • Multi-dose • Often inexpensive	• Difficult inhalation technique • Propellants required • High oropharyngeal deposition
pMDI + spacer device	
• Practical advantages as for pMDI • Easier to use effectively than pMDI • Reduced oropharyngeal deposition	• More bulky than pMDI • Propellants required • Susceptible to effects of static charge
DPI	
• Practical advantages similar to pMDI (if multidose or multiple single-dose) • No propellants needed • Inspiratory flow-actuated • Easier to use than pMDI	• Sometimes more costly than pMDI • Some may be moisture sensitive • Inspiratory flow-driven (potential problem at low inspiratory force)

Fig. 10.22. Some advantages and disadvantages of the three forms of portable inhaler.

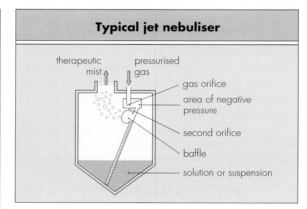

Typical jet nebuliser

Fig. 10.23. A typical jet nebuliser. The pressurised gas (air or oxygen) enters the chamber through a tube with a narrow orifice. A pressure drop causes the liquid to be sucked up from the reservoir and be broken into droplets. The larger of these fall back into the reservoir while the smaller droplets move with the stream of gas out of the nebuliser as a fine mist.

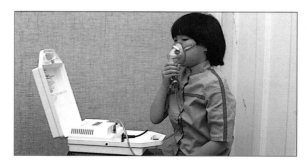

Fig. 10.24. Air compressor, nebuliser and face-mask in use by a child. The components of the system must be matched for performance characteristics.

11 COMPLEMENTARY TREATMENTS

Conventional treatment for asthma is usually both effective and free from significant adverse effects, and therefore health care professionals, particularly many doctors, often assume that the patient requires nothing else. There are, however, a number of other approaches to treatment which should be considered, either because they may be prescribed by medical practitioners or because patients may be recommended them by 'alternative practitioners'. Such complementary treatments range from the well-tested to the bizarre.

Many patients consult practitioners of complementary medicine without their doctor's knowledge, while others openly ask for alternative treatments. Pharmaceutical companies are subject to governmental controls on the efficacy and safety of their products, but alternative treatments are not subject to the same tight controls and with some of these treatments double-blind placebo-controlled studies are not possible. The lack of proven effectiveness means that such treatments should be viewed as 'complementary' not 'alternative', as 'alternative' implies that standard therapy can be discontinued or replaced by other treatments.

ALLERGEN AVOIDANCE

Most patients with asthma have a number of precipitating factors and cannot be treated successfully by avoidance of exposure to just one allergen. In a few cases, however, one trigger is dominant; and even if there are a number of obvious triggers, one may be particularly important and worth avoiding. The feasibility of avoidance depends upon the allergen, however.

- Several trials have now confirmed the efficacy of dust mite avoidance measures, although these are often difficult and/or costly to carry out. For example, the use of a mite-impermeable mattress cover for six weeks led to a 52% reduction in asthma symptoms in a group of mite-sensitive adults. Similar impermeable covers are available for duvets and pillows but these covers are much more costly than normal bedding materials. Various other methods of limiting exposure to dust mites and their faecal particles have been described (*see* **Fig 6.3**) but not all are effective or easy to apply.

- Pet cats are second only to house dust mites as a source of allergen responsible for perennial rhinitis (*see* **Fig. 16.19**). Removal of cats from the household, coupled with scrupulous cleaning of soft furnishings, is the definitive method of control for asthma associated with allergy to cats. Regular weekly washing of cats may lessen their allergic potential by removing dried saliva from their fur, and thus reducing the air-borne level of the principal allergen, the salivary protein *Fel d I*. If washing is combined with a reduction in soft furnishings and the removal of carpets, total allergen exposure is greatly reduced; so it may be possible, though not desirable, for cat-sensitive patients to live in a home containing cats.

- Allergy to dogs and other domestic animals is a less common cause of asthma but, ideally, patients should avoid contact with all animals to which they are allergic.

- It is difficult to avoid pollens completely but patients with pollen-sensitive asthma should keep the windows of cars and buildings closed during the pollen season, and avoid spending time in open spaces, especially in the evenings, when the pollen count is usually highest. Some cars and buildings have pollen-filtering air-conditioning systems, and personal filters are also available (**Fig. 11.1**), though they are inconvenient for regular use.

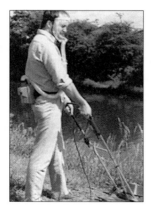

Fig. 11.1. Allergen avoidance; grass pollen. Grass pollen is difficult to avoid. Avoiding fields and freshly mown areas may help. Complete avoidance can be achieved by battery-powered respirators which filter the inspired air. Modern designs are relatively light and comfortable. Similar filters are included in some car and building air-conditioning systems.

- Occupational allergens may provoke severe and persistent asthma, which continues even in the absence of continued exposure, so early diagnosis and complete withdrawal from contact with the offending allergen are of particular importance. Early intervention in these patients may lead to a 'cure' of asthma. Withdrawal from allergen exposure is usually feasible in this situation, although this may cause employment problems for the patient. Sometimes, special equipment may prevent exposure to allergen in the workplace (**Fig. 11.2**).

DESENSITISATION

For many years there has been extensive interest in desensitisation schedules which aim to induce tolerance by gradually building up blocking antibodies. Unfortunately these regimes have shown little success in asthma and have been associated with local reactions and fatalities. The current recommendation in the UK is that desensitisation should only be carried out at sites where full resuscitation facilities are immediately available. It is possible that developments in desensitising therapy may lead to its greater use in the future.

PHYSICAL TREATMENTS

A number of different sorts of physical treatment have been advocated for asthma, although many have not been rigorously tested in a scientifically acceptable manner.

Breathing exercises attempt to teach a relaxed pattern of breathing during an attack, but there is little objective evidence to support their use. In episodes of mucus retention, physiotherapy can help expectoration.

General exercise and fitness are good for asthma. Although exercise provokes airway narrowing in many asthmatics, keeping fit is important because it will allow given tasks to be carried out with less overall ventilation. Swimming is a useful exercise in asthma because the saturated air being breathed is less likely to produce bronchoconstriction. Other helpful factors are an adequate warm-up before exertion and avoidance of very cold or foggy environments. A number of swimming exercise programmes now exist for asthmatic children. If necessary, adequate prophylactic medication should be taken beforehand. Many conventional asthma drugs are allowed under International Olympic and other regulations (*see* Chapter 18).

ACUPUNCTURE

This traditional Chinese form of complementary medicine relies on the 'readjusting of the balance of energies between organs' (**Fig. 11.3**) through needling meridians with acupuncture needles. The needles may also be electronically stimulated to increase their effectiveness. Acupuncture can be effective as an anaesthetic and pain reliever.

In asthma there is short-term evidence that following needling an exact point (Din Chuan point) on the back, respiratory function—PEF and FEV_1—can improve, with the degree of benefit being similar to the effects of a low dose of inhaled bronchodilator. Acupuncture a short distance away from this site has no effect on PEF. Similarly, both exercise-induced asthma and bronchial hyper-reactivity have been claimed to be reduced (although not blocked entirely) following a single acupuncture session, when compared with no acupuncture. However these studies were not adequately controlled.

Acupuncture is usually a repeated rather than a short-term treatment, but there is no evidence that long-term treatment is associated with any benefit. One study has suggested that long-term acupuncture can reduce the sensation of breathlessness but has no affect on airway calibre. Thus acupuncture alone could be potentially dangerous in reducing the patient's perception of the severity of their asthma. In China acupuncture is recommended to be linked with more traditional Western medicines and not used alone.

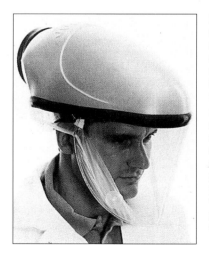

Fig. 11.2. Allergen avoidance; occupational asthma. A respirator with a filter is incorporated in the rigid hood. Although such devices are very effective in eliminating inhaled particles, they can prove difficult to work with in physically demanding jobs.

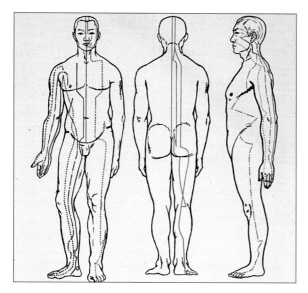

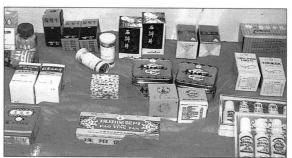

Fig. 11.4. Chinese herbal medicines. An array of Chinese herbal medicines on sale. These can be effective therapy as many contain biologically active naturally occurring ingredients such as ephedrine from the plant ephedra, a PAF antagonist from the ginkgo tree and naturally occurring steroid-like molecules. However, some unscrupulous herbalists add undeclared theophylline or steroids to ensure effect.

Fig. 11.3. Acupuncture. A model demonstrating the meridian lines and points for acupuncture. Needling the 'Din Chuan' point has been shown to lead to an improvement in respiratory function equivalent to the effect of a low dose of inhaled bronchodilators. Exercise-induced asthma may be reduced by acupuncture in the short term, but there are fears that acupuncture can reduce the sensation of breathlessness thus reducing the patient's awareness of the severity of asthma. In China, acupuncture is not recommended as a sole therapy and is usually accompanied by herbal and/or Western medicines.

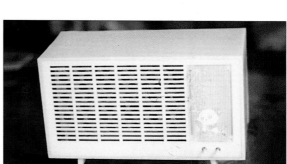

Fig. 11.5. Ionisers. Ionisers produce negatively charged particles to counteract positively charged ions which are thought to be associated with increase in asthma severity. Long-term use of such ionisers in the bedroom has not been shown to have any effect on asthmatics and is not recommended.

HERBAL MEDICINES

Herbal medicines and organic natural cures (**Fig. 11.4**) have been used for many centuries and in some cases are effective bronchodilators or may act as anti-inflammatory agents. The reason for this is that they are made from plants that contain active compounds, such as the ephedra plant which contains ephedrine, an effective bronchodilator, ginkgo tree extract, which has anti-PAF activity, and some plants containing high levels of naturally occurring steroid-like molecules. Drug doses contained in these preparations can vary widely and care must also be taken as some of the less scrupulous herbal medicine purveyors include in their herbal recipes pharmaceutically made methylxanthines and steroids to ensure efficacy, but do not warn the patient of the potential dangers.

IONISERS

Increases in breathlessness and asthma attacks are common when there are electrical storms or hot dry winds blowing. The associated high positive electrical charge at such times led to the idea that positively charged ions were asthmagenic and negatively charged ions therapeutic. Ionisers (**Fig. 11.5**) have been designed to generate increased quantities of negatively charged particles and in one study appeared to reduce long-term asthma symptoms in 10 of 11 children studied. However, all long-term studies, particularly those using ionisers in bedrooms, have shown no effect whatsoever on symptoms or frequency of attacks of asthma. Ionisers are ineffective and patients should be actively discouraged from wasting money on such devices.

HOMOEOPATHY

The central homoeopathic principle is 'like cures like' and the belief is that the remedy becomes more powerful the more dilute the solution becomes. As the solution is diluted, the diluting vessel is struck, thus imparting or allowing the process of 'succession' to take place, so however dilute the solution it is believed to carry information regarding the original substance. Unlike acupuncture, homoeopathy could be investigated using controlled trials, but these have not been performed in asthma. One study with a homoeopathic remedy in hay fever suggested a greater reduction in antihistamine use compared with placebo. However, no other studies have shown any effect in asthma, and homoeopathy is not recommended.

HYPNOSIS, RELAXATION AND YOGA

Acute attacks of asthma provoke anxiety and this itself can worsen asthma. A number of studies have demonstrated psychological effects on the airways; nebulised normal saline can induce bronchoconstriction or bronchodilatation according to the information given to the patient with the inhalation. It is therefore not surprising that relaxation techniques themselves or in association with other physical treatments may help asthmatics.

Hypnosis, in particular self-hypnosis, has been associated with reduced reactions to skin prick testing and can improve symptoms in chronic asthma. However, only a small percentage of asthmatics can be hypnotised successfully and very few can effectively self-hypnotise.

Relaxation exercises (**Fig. 11.6**) and yoga may reduce stress but no controlled studies have been carried out in asthma.

The use of these complementary techniques should not be associated with any reduction in preventive treatment without strict monitoring of symptoms and peak flow measurements at home.

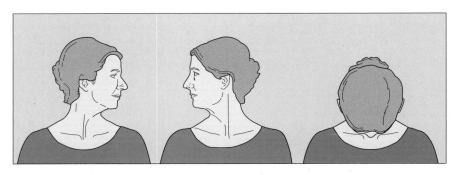

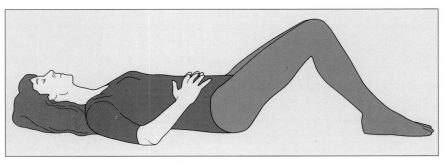

Fig. 11.6. Relaxation exercises. Relaxation exercises such as yoga are associated with a reduction in stress and, in a few patients, may reduce the need for rescue bronchodilators. Individual patients enjoy this type of treatment but reduction of preventive therapy should only be carried out in conjunction with symptom and PEF monitoring.

12 PATIENT EDUCATION

The increase in understanding of the pathogenesis of asthma with the introduction of effective and comparatively safe treatment regimens for the majority of patients should have led to a rapid and considerable reduction in morbidity and mortality from asthma. That this has not occurred may be associated with a change in severity and an increase in prevalence of asthma (*see* Chapter 1); but it may also be associated with patients failing to receive or follow appropriate medical advice. The changing relationship between doctors, other health professionals and patients over the past 25 years has meant that patients may wish to know more about their disease and treatment, and in many cases to be actively involved with their own management. Patients generally wish to be more 'empowered' and in control, particularly in a chronic disease with such a variable natural history as asthma.

Following the initial diagnosis of any chronic disease the patient is typically relieved at the making of a diagnosis, but also angry and likely to reject the diagnosis. At this time patients are unlikely to digest and recall all the information they receive, including simple information such as the timing and frequency of medication. It is essential to ensure that the patient's inhaler technique is adequate (**Figs 12.1–12.4**), and clear written instructions on medication and peak flow measurement, where appropriate, should be given to the patient (**Fig. 12.5**).

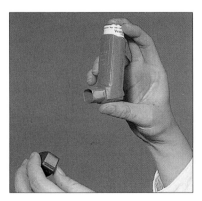

Figs 12.1–12.4. The manoeuvres involved in the co-ordinated use of a metered-dose inhaler.

Fig. 12.1. Remove cap and shake.

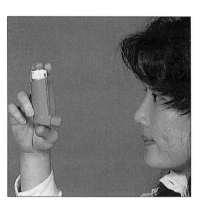

Fig. 12.2. Hold upright.

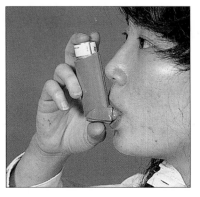

Fig. 12.3. Co-ordinate 'firing' and slow inspiration.

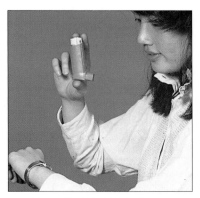

Fig. 12.4. Hold breath for at least 10 seconds.

The patient should be allowed time to ask questions about the disease, but initially may be unable to think of appropriate questions, and it is important to give further opportunities for questions on subsequent visits. The previously diagnosed asthmatic who is referred to a specialist clinic, or has been admitted to hospital with an acute attack of asthma, is usually more knowledgeable, but explanation of the disease process and personalised instruction is still important.

There is now a wide range of educational leaflets and audio and video cassettes explaining asthma medication, disease processes and avoidance measures (**Figs 12.6, 12.7**) which have been carefully designed, but not always evaluated for efficacy. This problem was highlighted by a study a number of years ago comparing two different education interventions in a controlled trial. One group received an education booklet about asthma (including advice on self-management), the other group received an audiotape to take home and had a short interview with the doctor, at which asthma information was given in a standard fashion. Both groups' knowledge of asthma increased, but there was no change in morbidity in either group. Knowledge of asthma does not appear to improve morbidity and, as a major component of this morbidity results from poor compliance, other educational programmes have been developed.

FOR NEXT 4 WEEKS

REGULAR — Brown inhaler (Pulmicort)
2 puffs morning & night
Rinse mouth and spit out after

AS NEEDED — Blue inhaler (Ventolin)
2 puffs when you need it

PEAK FLOW — Best of 3 blows morning and night

Bring diary card next time

Fig. 12.5. Handwritten information and instructions. Written instructions may be helpful, particularly soon after diagnosis and before the patient is able to be involved in a 'self-management' plan. Patients are often unable to remember all the advice, especially if they have just been diagnosed or their medication regimen is changed. The patient is also able to show written instructions to another health worker if there is a deterioration in their asthma.

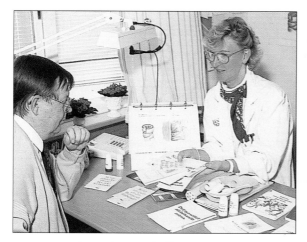

Fig. 12.6. Asthma education leaflets. An array of educational asthma leaflets is available in most countries, covering a wide range of specific topics related to the asthmatic, as well as giving an overall picture of asthma. Such leaflets can be used in conjunction with individualised written advice and medication instructions.

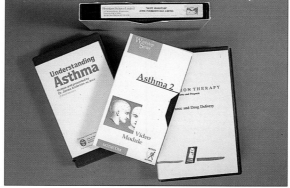

Fig. 12.7. Asthma education using audio and video cassettes. There is an increasing number of educational audio and video cassettes, some giving an overall view of asthma pathogenesis, treatment and problems, others focusing on a precise problem. Videos on inhaler technique, particularly those supplied with a checklist and for home loan, are effective. Asthma education audio tapes and video cassettes improve knowledge of asthma, but whether they improve morbidity without other intervention is not certain.

Booklets, cassette tapes and videos are excellent ways of imparting information about asthma, but are now recommended as part of an overall educational package and self-management plan, not as the sole approach to patient education.

COMPLIANCE WITH THERAPY

Compliance or *adherence* has been defined as the extent to which a person's behaviour (in terms of taking medications, following diets or executing life-style changes) coincides with medical or health advice. Compliance in asthma has not been extensively studied in the past, mainly because only indirect measurements were possible, such as patient reports, pill counts, inhaler weights or serum or urine drug levels (**Fig. 12.8**).

Drug containers may now be fitted with devices which record each time the container is opened. Studies in asthma have used the nebuliser chronolog (NC), which is attached to a pressurised metered dose inhaler (pMDI) (**Fig. 12.9**), and the Turbuhaler computer (TIC)

Assessment of therapeutic compliance	
Direct measurement of drug levels	
Blood	Single observation
Urine	Affected by patient preknowledge
Saliva	Not very quantitative
Indirect methods	
Patient interview	Inaccurate
Doctor belief	Very inaccurate
Pill counting	Not always applicable in asthma and bronchitis
Aerosol weighing, dry powder capsule counting/weighing	Not confirmed against direct measurement
Therapeutic outcome	Poor over long periods of time as the disease may fluctuate in severity

Fig. 12.8. Techniques used in the assessment of therapeutic compliance. Accurate estimation of compliance in asthma is now becoming possible with the introduction of electronic timed inhalers and diary cards. Previously, techniques were of limited value for the reasons shown here. Weighing of canisters is of limited value because of the small doses involved, and because of the possibility of multiple actuations to waste by the patient who knows compliance is being assessed. Similarly, semi-objective measurements, such as canister weighing and dose counting with Diskhaler and capsule inhalers, are limited by the possibility of patient wastage of doses (deliberate or accidental). Patient reports and physician assessment are also very poor indicators of compliance.

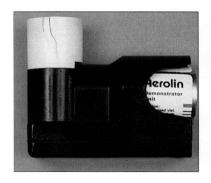
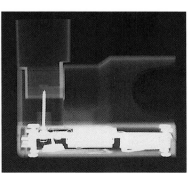

Fig. 12.9. Nebuliser chronolog. The first electronic recording device for identifying medication use with pMDI. The time of each actuation is recorded and can be obtained as a print out. Actuations very close to each other (just prior to a clinic visit) suggest drug 'dumping' by the patient. Drug dumping by test firing may occur recurrently and, as the device only records actuations, not inhalation, this will not be identified.

(**Fig. 12.10**), which is concealed inside the dry powder Turbuhaler (or Turbohaler). Both devices record the times the inhalers are activated.

Using the NC inhaler in a clinical trial, compliance with an inhaled anti-inflammatory was found to be disappointingly low on a four times daily regimen. Compliance was only good enough to make valid conclusions about the effect of the drug in six of the 24 patients. In another study, using the NC to look at bronchodilator use prescribed three times daily, 15% of patients were found to be using the inhalers as prescribed, while 14% of patients were observed to make multiple activations prior to clinic visits, interpreted as drug dumping.

A study of over 100 patients in mainly community practices used the TIC inhaler to compare compliance of a combination of β-agonist and inhaled steroid in a single inhaler and in two separate inhalers. This study also assessed anxiety and depression levels using the Hospital Anxiety Depression scale self ratings and a structured interview looking at health belief and other factors which could affect compliance, to see if non-compliant patients could be identified. The study ran for 12 weeks and medication was prescribed on a twice daily regimen, with patient care continued in the usual fashion either by general practitioner or practice nurse. Of the 100 patients, 30 failed to complete the study for a number of reasons (usually as the ultimate form of non-compliance). The results were disappointing overall with 40–50% of patients taking less than 80% of the prescribed medication; compliance with the combined inhaler was no better than with the separate inhalers (**Fig. 12.11**).

Apart from those few who followed the regimen almost perfectly, two patterns of drug taking emerged.

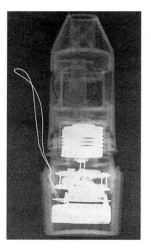

Fig. 12.10. Electronic recording dry powder inhaler (TIC). A radiograph of a modified multidose dry powder inhaler (Turbuhaler/Turbohaler). This incorporates a microphone which records the rotational click made to prime the device, and the noise of the inhalation. It stores the time of inhalation on a microchip. The data can be downloaded onto a computer to display the medication use of a patient and how this compares with the medical advice given by the physician.

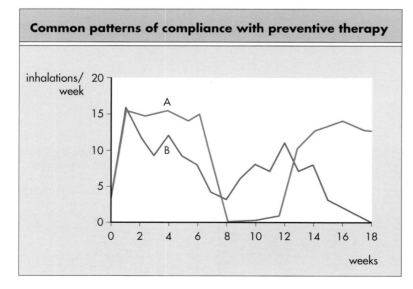

Fig. 12.11. Patterns of compliance, as studied using an electronic recording inhaler. Some patients are fully compliant, others very erratic in their inhaler use, but two patterns (shown here schematically) emerged in the moderately compliant patients:

A) Regular twice daily use for a few weeks following the physician's advice, then suddenly stopping and later resuming (presumably when symptoms returned). This 'holiday' type of pattern was not associated with severe exacerbations.

B) A sudden increase in medication use following a clinic visit, which falls away over the subsequent 6-week period. Earlier clinic 'scheduling' may prevent an exacerbation in some of these patients.

Psycho-social factors which may reduce compliance
• Depression
• Anxiety
• Denial of illness
• Shame
• Anger
• Isolation
• High-risk life style (smoking, alcohol abuse)

Fig. 12.12. Factors affecting compliance in patients with asthma.

One group showed high levels of compliance after the initiation of treatment followed by a slow decline, with an increase again following a clinic visit in mid-trial. The other group showed a pattern of regular compliance followed by stopping and resumption of therapy a few days or a week or so later.

The former pattern highlights the effectiveness of a clinic visit in reminding the patient of the need for medication and suggests that clinical scheduling could be a useful mechanism for improving compliance. The latter 'holiday' pattern suggests that as the patient feels better the perceived need for long term prophylactic treatment diminishes, but as symptoms return they act as a reminder to comply with the prescribed regimen.

There was a trend for older patients and those with longer duration since diagnosis to be more compliant. There was also a tendency for females to be less compliant. Anxiety levels were higher in females than in males and also in all patients than in normal individuals, but this did not lead to greater compliance. Depression was greater in the non-compliant population, however. There was a tendency for all patients to be both embarrassed and ashamed about their disease and for the more recently diagnosed to be angry and resentful (**Fig. 12.12**).

Although these studies have been useful in highlighting the pattern and complexity of poor compliance and showing that no single indicator identifies or helps the non-compliant patient, they may be subject to ethical criticism as the patients were not fully informed of the presence of the recording devices. However, a small study using an electromechanical device with patients on twice daily inhaled steroid therapy showed differences in behaviour between the fully informed group, who were told about the device, and the group who were not. These observations suggest that if a realistic measurement of compliance is to be made, the patients should be unaware that they are being monitored. Withholding such information has been considered justified as the studies carry minimal risk and do not adversely affect subjects' rights or welfare. When appropriate, patients have been given additional information after participation.

SELF-MANAGEMENT PLANS AND THE USE OF AT-HOME PEAK FLOW MONITORING

The introduction of inexpensive and simple peak flow meters has meant patients are able to monitor their degree of airflow obstruction and to correlate this with their symptoms. Regular at home PEF monitoring also allows the physician (and patient) to monitor the patient's response to changes in medication, environmental avoidance measures, or changes in life-style such as reducing cigarette consumption. The results may also reassure the doctor that he has made the correct diagnosis. Improvement in diary card scores in conjunction with improving PEF should reinforce, in the patient's eyes, the effectiveness of the doctor's advice. However, some patients have poor perception of the degree of severity of their asthma (*see* **Fig. 5.3**) and in some there is a lack of correlation with symptoms, such as breathlessness and nocturnal wakening. Not all patients are able and willing to carry out regular measurements of PEF, but for patients with severe asthma, or poor perception, such monitoring may not only be helpful but life saving. Studies using meters with electronic timing show that twice daily measurement with memory aids can be associated with a high degree of compliance, but some patients still fail to record the time accurately, or will generate false data to please the physician.

Self-management plans focus on the early recognition of deteriorating asthma using PEF recordings and/or symptoms. Written guidelines are individually developed

Example of management plan*	
Potential normal PEF†	550 l/min
Routine treatment	Becloforte inhaler‡ 1 puff 2 × day Ventolin (salbutamol) inhaler 1 puff 2 × day and when required
PEF < 400 l/min	Increase Becloforte to 1 puff 4 × day and Ventolin (salbutamol) to 1–2 puffs 4 × day and when required
PEF < 250 l/min	Prednisolone 40mg/day until PEF > 500 l/min, then prednisolone 20mg/day for same number of days
PEF < 150 l/min	Contact general practitioner urgently or go to hospital emergency department

*Example of written management plan given to male patient aged 39 years
†Predicted peak expiratory flow (PEF) = 540, best consistent PEF 550 l/min
‡Beclamethosone dipropionate inhaler, 250µg/actuation

Fig. 12.13. Self-management guidelines using at-home PEF monitoring. PEF measurement at home with written guidelines should reduce asthma morbidity and this early example was shown to be effective. However, the complexity of these guidelines limits their general use and they have been superseded by simple but equally effective guidelines using a 'credit card' plan.

so that, as the patient's symptoms worsen or (after an exacerbation) improve, they are able to adjust therapy or obtain medical assistance appropriately (**Fig. 12.13**).

Initial guidelines were based on the educational value of PEF monitoring for patients (**Fig. 12.14**), but these plans were complicated (**Fig. 12.13**). An open study showed improvement in retrospective and cross-sectional measures of severity. A PEF self-management plan using a simple interpretation of PEF with colour coding of the worsening of the patient's asthma rather than precise changes of PEF (**Fig. 12.15**) was associated with similar improvements in morbidity. In both studies other education and support were provided, making it difficult to decide which specific features were most effective.

Symptom-based self-management plans have also been shown to be effective in most patients. A recent study using a 'credit card' asthma self-management plan compared PEF and symptoms in a community care study in New Zealand (**Fig. 12.16**). The 'credit card' plan consisted of a plastic card with written guidelines for the self-management of asthma. On one side the guidelines were based on the interpretation of PEF recordings, whilst those on the reverse were symptom based. The introduction of the 'credit card' was associated with a significant reduction in asthma morbidity, with a halving of nights woken and days 'out of action' due to asthma.

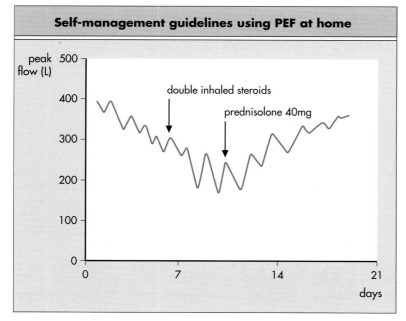

Self-management guidelines using PEF at home

peak flow (L)

double inhaled steroids

prednisolone 40mg

days

Fig. 12.14. Self-management guidelines using PEF monitoring at home. Monitoring PEF at home with written guidelines on changes in medication may avoid acute hospitalisation, as shown here. Following the development of a sore throat the patient noted a fall in PEF and responded by doubling the dose of inhaled steroids. There was no improvement in his PEF, which in fact fell further and the patient developed nocturnal wakening. In accordance with his guidelines the patient started prednisolone, 40 mg each morning, which was associated with improvement in his PEF. He maintained his higher dose of inhaled steroids and completed his 10-day course of oral steroids. His peak flow was well maintained over the following week and he returned to his normal daily dose of inhaled steroids, having avoided a severe attack or hospitalisation.

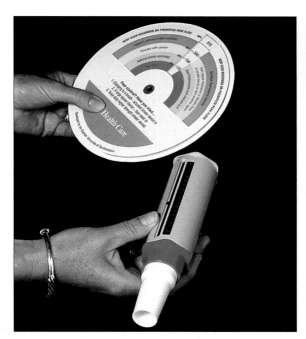

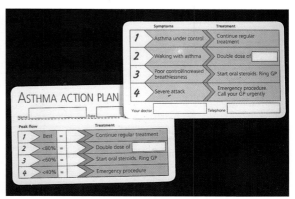

12.16. 'Credit card' self-management guidelines. The
credit card plan consists of written guidelines for the self-assessment of asthma printed on a plastic card. On one side management guidelines are based on the interpretation of PEF recordings and on the reverse they are based on symptoms. The introduction of this self-management plan was associated with a significant reduction in asthma mortality. Of the subjects, 28% found the PEF more helpful in an exacerbation of asthma, and 7% found symptoms more helpful, while the majority (48%) found both sides of the card equally helpful. (D'Souza, *Eur Respir J* 1994; **7**: 1260–5.)

Fig. 12.15. Self-management using at-home PEF measurement with a colour coding device.

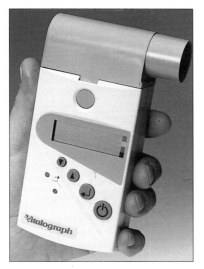

Fig. 12.17. Electronic diary card with interactive self-management programmes.
An electronic diary card with an integrated peak flow meter which can be programmed for an individual patient's predicted PEF and percentage predicted PEF is under investigation. The diary card has a real-time clock so the patient can be reminded by an alarm to measure peak flow. The message display asks the patients about their symptoms and prompts them to take their medication. Falling PEFs are assessed and the patient is then instructed to increase their inhaled steroids, take a course of oral steroids or seek medical assistance. Improving PEFs will be associated with instructions to reduce treatment. The cost effectiveness of such an interactive computer programme is still being investigated, but with the increasing acceptance of computer technology and falling costs this option may be useful in the future for some severe asthmatics.

An interesting research approach to self-management plans is the introduction of an electronic diary card (**Fig. 12.17**) with integral computer programme and a 'scrolling' text. An electronic peak flow meter is built into the diary card, together with a real time clock which can be programmed to give an 'alarm' signal at different times to remind the patient to measure PEF. The diary card has a text window which asks the patient to record symptoms and to take prescribed medication. The programmable diary card can be 'tailored' to the individual patient's PEF, so percent predicted or percent best-ever PEF can be entered. Changes in PEF or symptoms will prompt instructions for the patient to increase the dose of inhaled steroid, take a course of oral steroids, seek medical advice, or step down treatment appropriately. Although only at the research stage, such devices, if shown to be effective, may have a place in the management of asthma.

THE PRACTICE NURSE

There is increasing awareness of the need for a multi-disciplinary approach in delivering health care to asthmatic patients.

The role of specialist asthma clinics in hospitals and the community is now well established, but nurse practitioners or practice nurses must be trained appropriately. Training for nurses to run asthma clinics has been available in the UK and USA for some years. Distance-learning courses, using informative material, case studies and in-course assessment, are an initial way but additional residential courses are desirable. The National Asthma Training Centre in the UK is an example (**Fig. 12.18**) where nurses attend an intensive residential course on all aspects of asthma, not only PEF and inhaler use, but also behavioural educational training and communication skills. Initial videos and interviews with feedback highlight the nurses' initial tendency to be concerned (like doctors) with the straightforward tasks of writing instructions and demonstrating inhalers, and to lose sight of the patients' needs or difficulties following such instructions. When trained, nurses may be in a better position not only to obtain more medical information but, more importantly, to alter the social and economic pressures on the patient. Patients may seemingly be unwilling to waste a doctor's time on such apparently unimportant or unrelated details, but may inform the nurse of such matters.

A well-run asthma clinic requires adherence to a check list to ensure the patient's asthma is under control, inhaler technique is correct, and potential problems such as holidays abroad are dealt with. Bone density assessment should be arranged for perimenopausal asthmatics on high dose inhaled steroids and/or intermittent oral steroids. A more 'open ended' element is also required so that personal and family problems which affect asthma can be brought out. A rigid 'check list' alone is inadequate.

EDUCATIONAL PROGRAMMES

Integrated educational programmes including verbal and written personal instructions, pamphlets, and audio and video cassettes are effective at imparting information. Group discussions with other asthmatics, exercise programmes and behavioural games are also helpful in decreasing morbidity.

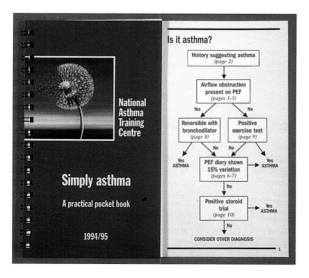

Fig. 12.18. Training asthma nurses. At an asthma training centre in the UK, hospital nurse practitioners and practice nurses may enter a 'distant' training course on asthma, followed by a residential course covering additional aspects of asthma medication and communication/interview skills. Specialist asthma clinics in the community are an important development in the multidisciplinary approach to the treatment of asthma, and appropriate training of all staff is essential.

13 NATURAL HISTORY OF CHILDHOOD ASTHMA

Asthma is the commonest chronic disease of children and adolescents, and childhood asthma has become one of the major health problems in most developed countries around the world. It is the most frequent chronic disease to cause absence from school, and it has a profound effect on long-term health and scholastic attainment, thus affecting many children for the rest of their lives.

EPIDEMIOLOGY

There is considerable evidence of an increase in prevalence and severity of asthma in childhood in most developed countries. Thus, one study in South Wales showed an increase in the point prevalence of asthma in 12-year-old children from 4% in 1973 to 9% in 1988 (**Fig. 13.1**; *see also* **Fig. 1.8**), using identical diagnostic criteria at each phase. This study also identified increases in eczema from 8 to 14% and hay fever from 3 to 8% over the same period (**Fig. 13.1**). Similar observations have been made elsewhere in Europe, Australia, New Zealand and Taiwan.

Prevalence figures for current asthma in mid-childhood range from 5.4% in the United States to 16% in England and 25% in Australia. The life-time prevalence rates for asthma reach 32% in Australia. There has also been a very considerable increase in hospital admissions for childhood asthma over the past 8–10 years with no reduction in severity on admission, no increase in re-admission ratios and no evidence of significant diagnostic transfer (*see* Chapter 1).

ASTHMA DEATHS IN CHILDHOOD

Death from asthma in childhood is rare: 40–45 children die each year in England and Wales from the disease. There has been a steady diminution in mortality rates in the 0–4-year-old group, but no change between the ages of 5–14 years. During the mid-1960s, there was an increase in mortality in the 10–14-year-old group, which

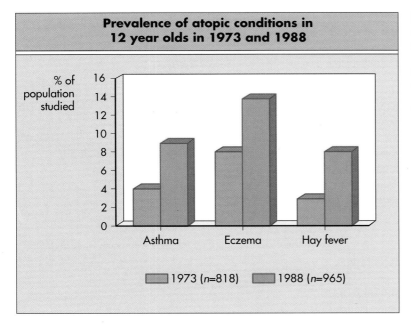

Fig. 13.1. The point prevalence of atopic conditions in 12-year-old children in South Wales in 1973 and 1988. Asthma, eczema and hay fever commonly co-exist, and all three conditions showed a significant increase in prevalence over the 15-year period (Burr *et al.*, *Arch Dis Child* 1989;**64**:1452–6).

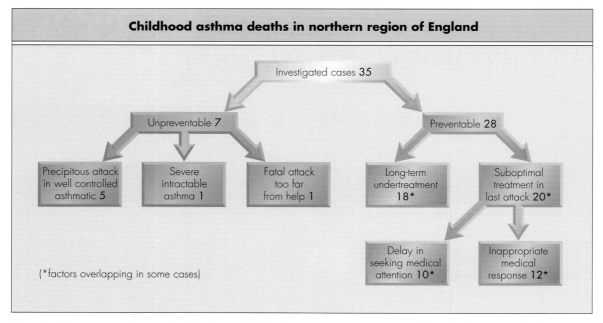

Childhood asthma deaths in northern region of England

Investigated cases **35**

Unpreventable **7**

Preventable **28**

Precipitous attack in well controlled asthmatic **5**

Severe intractable asthma **1**

Fatal attack too far from help **1**

Long-term undertreatment **18***

Suboptimal treatment in last attack **20***

Delay in seeking medical attention **10***

Inappropriate medical response **12***

(*factors overlapping in some cases)

Fig. 13.2. The outcome of an audit of deaths in childhood asthma in Northern England. Most asthma deaths were judged to have been potentially preventable, and the commonest underlying causes related to sub-optimal long-term or acute treatment. Nevertheless, some deaths in childhood may be totally unpredictable and therefore essentially unavoidable (Fletcher *et al., Arch Dis Child* 1990;**65**:163–7).

paralleled the increase in adult asthma deaths. The cause of this epidemic has been discussed at length but even today remains unresolved, although it may relate to the inappropriate use of bronchodilators rather than anti-inflammatory prophylactic compounds (*see* Chapter 1). A similar explanation has been suggested for the more recent epidemic of asthma deaths in New Zealand which was associated with the regular use of high potency inhaled β-agonists.

Studies in children who have died of asthma have suggested similar predisposing factors to those in adults, including delayed treatment in the final attack, adverse psycho-social factors, poor perception of air flow limitation and severe bronchial hyperresponsiveness. Whilst most asthma deaths are potentially preventable, there is a suggestion that some deaths in childhood may be totally unpredictable and therefore unavoidable (**Fig. 13.2**).

INFANTILE WHEEZE AND ASTHMA

Wheezing in infancy (**Fig. 13.3**) is a common problem, but does not always indicate an underlying diagnosis of asthma (*see* Chapter 14). Allergy is the most important factor in predicting the persistence and severity of wheezing in childhood. Isolated wheezing episodes in infancy have a poor predictive value for continuing

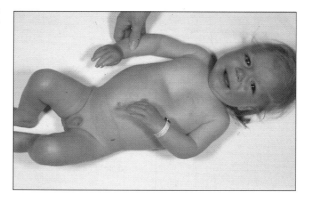

Fig. 13.3. A 13-month-old boy with acute wheezing. This picture demonstrates typical indrawing of the lower sternum. Infants have a very compliant chest wall which is easily deformed during respiratory distress, facilitating the collapse of the small airways. Permanent chest deformity may result from repeated episodes of wheezing.

asthma at the ages of 5 and 10 years. Only 15–20% of infant wheezers continue to have asthma in later childhood.

There are two main categories of infant wheezers:

- Most wheezy infants have transient episodes of wheeze, predominantly associated with viral infections. In this group wheezing usually remits by the age of 3 or 4 years. Predisposing factors include maternal smoking during pregnancy, low birth weight and chronic lung disease of prematurity. In this group it seems likely that intermittent symptomatic therapy is adequate management, as long-term sequelae are unusual.

- In some infants, wheezing is associated with atopy, which may not be manifest in other ways until the child is older. This form of wheezing is far more likely to represent true asthma, to persist, and to require long-term prophylactic therapy.

It is often difficult to distinguish which category an infant falls into, which makes decisions about therapeutic intervention difficult. The presence of eosinophilic inflammation in the airways is probably diagnostic of asthma and predictive of ongoing problems (see Chapter 2), but this cannot currently be detected in a non-invasive manner.

There is increasing evidence that environmental factors in fetal or early life lead to the development of an allergic constitution and thus to asthma. Possible factors are summarised in **Fig. 13.4**. Some of these factors are avoidable or preventable, while others may respond to appropriate therapeutic measures. Early intervention with prophylactic therapy is likely to be a valuable strategy for preventing ongoing disease, but this has yet to be conclusively demonstrated.

NATURAL HISTORY OF CHILDHOOD ASTHMA

Many paediatric textbooks state that childhood asthma is usually a self-limiting disorder which improves spontaneously during adolescence. This is misleading and inaccurate. Whilst mild episodic asthma of mid-childhood is predominantly self-limiting, those children with more persistent or chronic disease rarely experience remission. Prognosis is less favourable in children with an early age of onset, frequent or prolonged attacks in the first year after onset and associated atopic disease such as infantile eczema.

The male to female ratio is 1:1 for mild episodic asthma in childhood, but 4:1 in children with chronic severe asthma. As severe adult asthma has a sex ratio close to 1:1, it is likely that more males improve or remit in adolescence, whilst more females have persistent problems or develop more severe asthma during adolescence. The only factor known to be associated with a decreased probability of improvement in asthma symptoms amongst patients who have wheezed since early childhood is smoking in adolescence.

Currently there is no evidence that treatment can 'cure' childhood asthma. The early use of inhaled

Possible risk factors for wheezing in infancy
Prenatal
• Poor fetal nutrition – reduced airway diameter • Parental atopy • Maternal smoking • Maternal exposure to other pollutants or allergens • Materno-fetal immunological priming
Postnatal
• High exposure to allergens in early life • Virus infections • Tobacco smoke • Possibly other environmental pollutants

Fig. 13.4. Possible risk factors for wheezing in infancy.

steroids in childhood asthma has been shown to lead to improvement in lung function (**Fig. 13.5**) and bronchial hyperresponsiveness when compared with the use of inhaled β_2-agonist alone (as in adults; *see* Chapter 16). Such anti-inflammatory therapy is beneficial in suppressing symptoms and preventing deterioration and permanent damage, but it is not curative. Relapse remains a common problem if inhaled steroid therapy is reduced to too low a level or stopped.

PATHOPHYSIOLOGY

In adults, there is clear evidence that asthma is associated with airway inflammation in which eosinophils and mast cells play a prominent role (*see* Chapter 2). This has not yet been investigated in children below the age

of 5, although in older children evidence is accumulating to support the role of similar pathological processes to those in adults.

Transient wheezing of infancy associated with viral infections is probably not associated with persistent airway inflammation. The airway calibre of infants is small, their compliant chest walls allow the airways to collapse towards the end of expiration, and this tendency may be exacerbated by poor fetal lung growth. It disappears during normal growth in childhood. It is probably only those infants that develop inflammation who will have ongoing disease. The establishment of non-invasive markers for eosinophilic inflammation in the future may allow the identification of infants in this category at an early age, and thus provide the opportunity for early and effective therapeutic intervention.

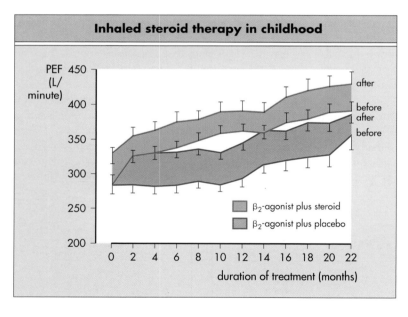

Fig. 13.5. Anti-inflammatory therapy with inhaled steroid (budesonide) is more effective than treatment with β_2-agonist (salbutamol) alone in childhood asthma. In this Dutch study, mean morning PEF, before and after bronchodilator (salbutamol, 200 µg) was monitored in two matched groups of children (aged 7–16 years). Only data from patients remaining in the trial are included in the analysis at each stage. This underestimates the difference between the two groups, as the cumulative withdrawal rate because of inadequate control in the group receiving β_2-agonist alone was 45%, while that in the steroid-treated group was just 5% (van Essen-Zandvliet et al., *Am Rev Respir Dis* 1992; **146**: 547–54).

14 CLINICAL FEATURES OF CHILDHOOD ASTHMA

HISTORY

Childhood asthma is characterised by episodes of paroxysmal coughing, particularly at night. Indeed, this is quite frequently the only presenting symptom in younger children. Sensations of chest tightness, breathlessness and wheezing become more obvious in mid-childhood.

Acute exacerbations of asthma in childhood are frequently associated with an upper respiratory tract viral infection, but may be triggered by exercise, particularly outdoors in cold or dry weather, emotional disturbance, laughing and exposure to allergens or non-specific irritants. There may be a seasonal variation in symptoms and it is particularly common to find a diurnal variation in symptoms, with night waking and severe symptoms on rising in the morning.

Children who present with frequent apparent respiratory infections, or who have persistent coughing lasting for weeks after a viral infection, are likely to have asthma. Most will respond better to anti-asthma therapy than to antibiotics. Those few patients who have genuine recurrent bacterial respiratory infections usually have another underlying disease such as cystic fibrosis,

ciliary dyskinesia syndrome or immune deficiency. Such children may also present with wheezing, but this is usually different in nature from the wheezing of asthma (*see* page 84).

In taking a history, it is important to enquire about the induction of symptoms by exposure to allergens, including pets, and by physical factors such as changes in temperature, humidity or exposure to tobacco smoke. As in adults, house dust mite is the commonest allergen and the type of housing is important. Such factors as the age of the property, its proximity to water, type of heating, carpeting, furniture and bedding may be important in relation to house dust mite colonisation. Soft toys can be a particularly important reservoir of house mites. Children spend about 12 hours per day in the bedroom, so details of bedding and furnishings may be important (**Fig. 14.1**).

In schoolchildren there may be additional problems related to the classroom. These may contain pets or plants. Furthermore, significant concentrations of dust mite, cat and dog allergens are brought into schools on the clothing of other children, and this can sometimes be a problem.

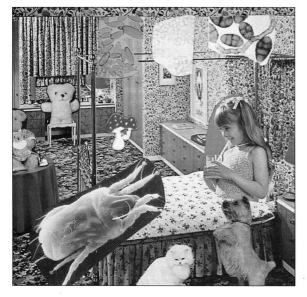

Fig. 14.1. A collage of the allergens which commonly affect children. These include house dust mite, animal saliva and danders, pollens, moulds and foods. The principal reservoirs of the house dust mite (*Dermatophagoides pteronyssinus* is shown in the scanning electron micrograph) are soft furnishings, including carpets and curtains, and stuffed toys.

The clinical history should include questions on associated atopic problems such as eczema, rhinitis, conjunctivitis, urticaria, angioedema and food intolerance. The history of pregnancy, birth and immediate postnatal period may provide information on predisposing factors related to transient wheezing of infancy or atopic asthma.

Of children with atopic asthma, 80% have at least one first degree relative with atopic problems, so a detailed family history is important. The smoking habits of the parents and their occupations may also have an impact on the child's disease.

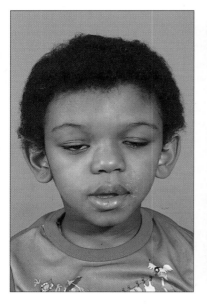

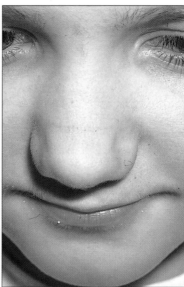

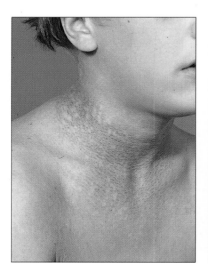

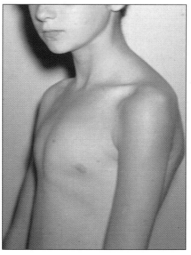

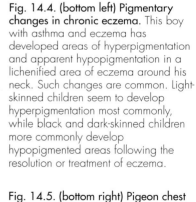

Fig. 14.2. (top left) A 7-year-old boy with asthma. He has characteristic atopic facies, with a lethargic expression, infraorbital and perioral oedema, a swollen and congested nose and some facial eczema, especially around his mouth.

Fig. 14.3. (top right) A pigmented transverse nasal crease resulting from repeated upward rubbing of the nose in allergic rhinitis (the 'allergic salute'). This 10-year-old girl with perennial rhinitis had been rubbing her nose upwards with the palm of her hand regularly for several years. Note the oedematous enlargement of the bridge of the nose and upper cheeks, commonly associated with chronic rhinitis.

Fig. 14.4. (bottom left) Pigmentary changes in chronic eczema. This boy with asthma and eczema has developed areas of hyperpigmentation and apparent hypopigmentation in a lichenified area of eczema around his neck. Such changes are common. Light-skinned children seem to develop hyperpigmentation most commonly, while black and dark-skinned children more commonly develop hypopigmented areas following the resolution or treatment of eczema.

Fig. 14.5. (bottom right) Pigeon chest (pectus carinatum) in a 10-year-old girl with asthma. Her asthma has been poorly controlled throughout childhood The sternum and costochondral junctions form a prominent ridge in the anterior chest, and the ribs slope away steeply to either side. Pigeon chest is usually a manifestation of the impact of chronic hyperinflation of the chest on growth in childhood.

EXAMINATION

The stigmata of allergic disease are often present. A typical allergic facies is often described, and is particularly common in children with associated rhinitis and eczema. Typically, there are discoloured swollen eyelids ('allergic shiners') and signs of mouth breathing (**Fig. 14.2**), and there may be a transverse nasal crease, because of a constant nose rubbing (**Fig. 14.3**). Serous otitis media with conductive deafness and allergic conjunctivitis may also be found. Atopic eczema occurs in at least 50% of children with asthma, and it may be obvious and active (*see* **Figs 1.14, 5.6**), or quiescent but associated with areas of depigmentation, hyperpigmentation or chronic lichenification (**Fig. 14.4**).

Children have a highly compliant thoracic cage (*see* **Fig. 13.3**). They, therefore, quite commonly develop chest deformity with either pectus excavatum or carinatum (**Fig. 14.5**) associated with Harrison's sulci (**Fig. 14.6**) and even a slight degree of spinal kyphosis with more severe disease. Those with severe problems may be underweight and growth delayed. Puberty can be markedly delayed in children with poorly managed asthma, although most children ultimately achieve relatively normal adult height. It is important to make accurate measurements of height and weight and plot these on appropriate centile charts (**Fig. 14.7**).

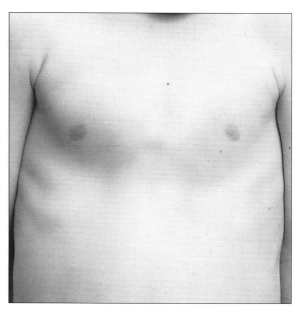

Fig. 14.6. Harrison's sulci in an 8-year old boy who had poorly treated asthma since the age of 2 years. The sulci are horizontal grooves on each side of the chest, several rib spaces wide. They are thought to occur as a result of traction of the diaphragms on the lower ribs during episodes of wheezing.

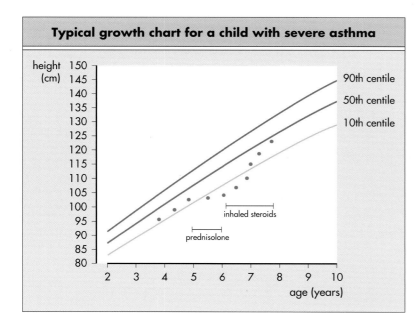

Fig. 14.7. Typical growth chart for a child with severe asthma. When first diagnosed the child was on the 15th centile. His uncontrolled asthma was subsequently treated with a prolonged course of oral prednisolone therapy, during which his growth was significantly impaired. Later he was weaned onto inhaled steroid therapy while maintaining control of his asthma. At this stage catch-up growth was seen, and he approached the 50th centile.

DIFFERENTIAL DIAGNOSIS AND INVESTIGATIONS

The clinical history should identify most patients with an alternative cause for wheezing (**Fig. 14.8**). A neonatal onset of symptoms, associated failure to thrive, evidence of bacterial infection, vomiting and choking in association with respiratory symptoms, focal lung or cardiovascular signs, or a monophonic rather than polyphonic wheeze, all suggest alternative diagnoses.

The nature of the wheeze may help to establish the diagnosis (**Fig. 14.9**). Monophonic wheezing is usually associated with a fixed obstruction in a large airway such as an inhaled foreign body (*see* **Figs 8.10, 8.11**), bronchomalacia, bronchogenic cyst or primary tuberculosis. Polyphonic wheeze may occur in association with cystic fibrosis (*see* **Figs 8.4, 8.5**), recurrent milk aspiration, primary ciliary dyskinesia syndrome or immune deficiency with recurrent infection.

A chest radiograph should be performed in most children with suspected asthma to exclude alternative diagnoses, but in most cases the chest film will be normal or show only nonspecific changes in patients who have asthma (**Fig. 14.10**). More severe changes may be seen in children with chronic undiagnosed or uncontrolled asthma (**Fig. 14.11**).

Beyond the chest radiograph, other investigations may be indicated by the clinical history and findings on examination. These may include:
- A Mantoux test for tuberculosis.
- A sweat test for cystic fibrosis.
- Immune function measurements if immune deficiency is suspected
- Reflux studies for aspiration.
- Studies of ciliary function.

Clinical features which help to distinguish between asthma and alternative diagnoses	
Suggestive of asthma	Suggestive of an alternative diagnosis
Wheeze and/or cough which is:	Neonatal onset
episodic	Failure to thrive
nocturnal	Chronic infection
seasonal	Vomiting with choking
exercise-induced	Focal lung signs
Associated atopic features, e.g. eczema	Cardiovascular signs
Family history of atopy	Monophonic wheeze

Fig. 14.8. Clinical features which help to distinguish between asthma and alternative diagnoses.

Differential diagnosis of wheezing in infancy
Asthma
Bronchiolitis (post respiratory syncytial virus syndrome)
Others

Monophonic wheeze

Inhaled foreign body
Vascular ring
Bronchogenic cyst
Enteric duplication cyst
Primary tuberculosis
Localised bronchomalacia

Polyphonic wheeze

Milk aspiration
Cystic fibrosis
Immune deficiency
Primary ciliary dyskinesia syndrome
Williams Campbell syndrome

Fig. 14.9. Differential diagnosis of wheezing in infancy.

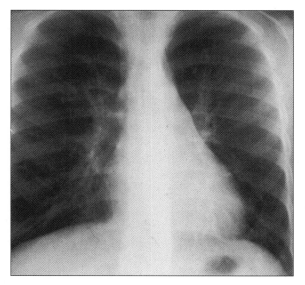

Fig. 14.10. Postero-anterior chest radiograph from a 10-year-old girl with asthma, demonstrating hyperinflation of the lung fields. This can be assessed by counting the anterior ends of the ribs above the mid-diaphragmatic point on the right. Normally, five ribs can be seen clear of the diaphragm, but in this film there are seven. The film also demonstrates peribronchial thickening with tramline shadows radiating away from both hila. These changes are consistent with a diagnosis of asthma, but they are not specific to it.

In children where the history is suggestive of asthma, frequent measurements of PEF (*see* **Figs 4.5, 4.6, 14.12**), and monitoring of lung function and of bronchodilator responsiveness after provocation testing (usually by exercise; **Figs 14.13, 14. 14**), may highlight the problem. Skin prick tests with a small range of allergens may help to identify atopic children (*see* **Figs 7.10, 7.11**). Children who produce sputum during attacks may be a cause of particular confusion, and cytology of the sputum to identify eosinophils or eosinophil proteins may be helpful here (*see* **Fig. 7.3**).

Lung function tests cannot, of course, be performed in infants and uncooperative children. If there is still doubt about the diagnosis in these patients, a diagnostic trial of anti-asthma therapy is often the most practical way to confirm the diagnosis.

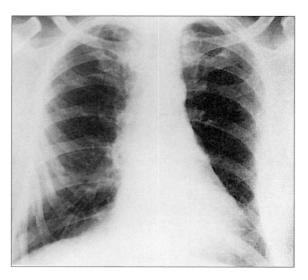

Fig. 14.11. Rib deformity from chronic childhood asthma. Prolonged uncontrolled asthma in children may result in a persistent rib cage deformity, There is indrawing of the lower ribs produced by the action of the flattened diaphragm in the chronically overinflated chest and the appearance of the right lower zone suggests the presence of bronchial wall thickening.

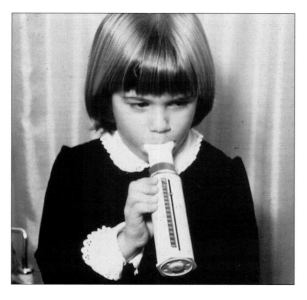

Fig. 14.12. A 4-year-old girl using a Wright Mini Peak Flow Meter. Most children over the age of 4 years can achieve reproducible results, and regular measurement of PEF facilitates the monitoring of asthma, at home and in the clinical setting.

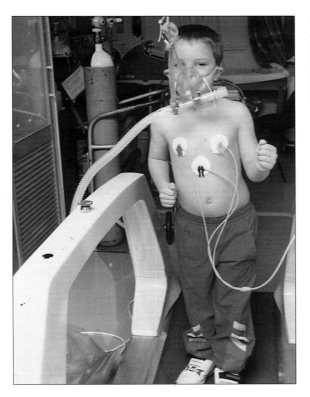

Fig. 14.13. A 6-year-old child undertaking a formal exercise test in an exercise laboratory. He is running on a treadmill and is breathing cold dry air which will enhance the exercise-induced response. An ECG monitor is also attached. Care should be taken in this test, as exhausted small children may be thrown back off the treadmill with some force.

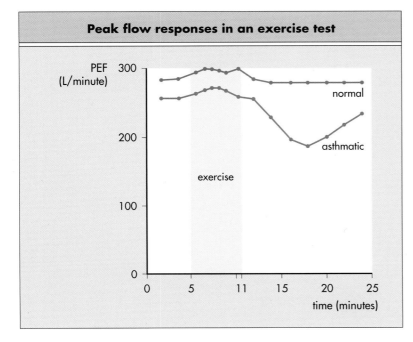

Fig. 14.14. The PEF response to exercise testing in a child. In normal subjects there is a small degree of bronchodilatation, and thus an increase in PEF, during exercise. In patients with asthma this initial bronchodilatation is followed by bronchoconstriction, which reaches its maximum 5–10 minutes after the end of exercise. A 15% drop from baseline level of PEF is considered a positive exercise test. Once this level is reached, the reversibility of the bronchoconstriction can be confirmed by the administration of an inhaled bronchodilator.

The processes which may lead to a diagnosis of asthma in a child are summarised in **Fig. 14.15**.

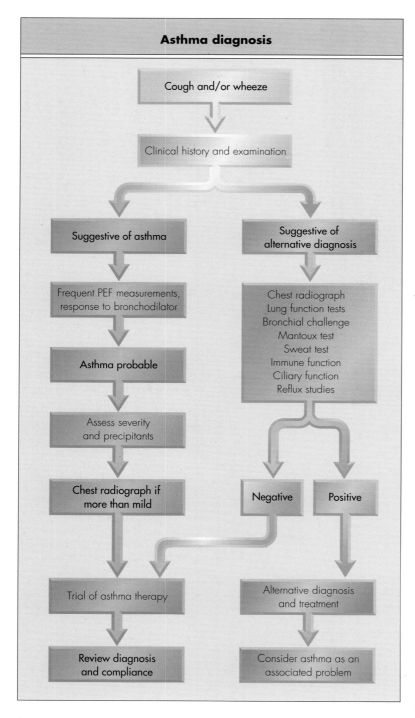

Fig. 14.15. A diagnostic algorithm for the child with recurrent cough and wheeze. Fig. 14.9 lists those features suggestive of asthma or suggestive of an alternative diagnosis and allows the diagnostic progress as outlined on this algorithm to be followed. This algorithm is taken from the Paediatric Asthma Consensus publication: Warner *et al.*, *Arch Dis Child* 1992;**67**:240–8.

15 MANAGEMENT OF CHILDHOOD ASTHMA

The goals of asthma management in childhood are to achieve resolution of any acute symptoms and then to use prophylactic drugs to reduce long-term morbidity. Such treatment should prevent exercise-induced symptoms and acute exacerbations associated with infection, and should allow the child to lead a normal existence.

The new understanding of the pathophysiology of established asthma in childhood implies that drugs which have a beneficial effect on the underlying eosinophilic airway inflammation are likely to be the most effective form of prophylaxis in childhood, as in adult asthma. Long-term follow-up studies to support or refute this view are in progress, and there is already a clear consensus in favour of widespread and early use of anti-inflammatory disease-modifying agents. Sodium cromoglycate has a useful in children with mild to moderate disease, but in more severe disease the major form of anti-inflammatory therapy in childhood, as in adult asthma, is inhaled steroid therapy.

GENERAL MEASURES

Environmental modification can have major beneficial effects, and in an ideal environment the requirement for conventional pharmacotherapy diminishes appreciably. This has been demonstrated in children moved to institutions at high altitude where exposure to allergens, and cigarette smoke and other pollutants, is appreciably reduced. Even children with severe disease are nearly always able to stop all regular asthma prophylaxis whilst still achieving considerable improvement in all parameters of disease severity. At present, it is not possible to recreate such an environment within the normal home without considerable extra expenditure, but three approaches should always be considered:

- Parents should be strongly encouraged to stop smoking and to make the home a smoke-free zone.
- Pets should usually be excluded from the home. Regular washing of cats may reduce the load of salivary allergen in the fur, but is usually less practicable and effective than complete exclusion. Pets should never be allowed in the child's bedroom.

- Dust mite control measures have varying degrees of efficacy (*see* **Fig. 6.3**) and may be helpful. Allergen avoidance is further discussed in Chapter 6.

MILD EPISODIC ASTHMA

Children with mild episodic asthma grow normally, miss little schooling and have minimal or no lung function abnormality between attacks. Inhaled β_2-agonists, used for short periods during attacks, are often the only necessary form of drug therapy. Where children develop exercise-induced asthma, a dose of inhaled bronchodilator immediately before exercise is protective in most cases. In infant wheezers, and in children whose asthma is accompanied by allergic rhinitis, non-sedating antihistamines (selective H_1-antagonists) may have some value as first stage prophylaxis.

FREQUENT EPISODIC ASTHMA

Where attacks are more frequent, prophylactic anti-inflammatory therapy is always required. The International Paediatric Asthma Consensus Group recommends that whenever a child needs more than three doses of bronchodilator per week, anti-inflammatory therapy should be started.

Clinical experience suggests that sodium cromoglycate has a useful prophylactic effect in up to 60% of children with mild-to-moderate seasonal or perennial asthma. Its duration of action is approximately 4 hours and it must be administered by inhaler at least three or four times daily. It is also often helpful where asthmatic attacks are triggered by exercise, cold air or allergen exposure, and where cough is the predominant symptom. Significant side effects are extremely rare. It may be necessary to add periodic bronchodilator therapy if the child experiences breakthrough symptoms.

Inhaled steroid therapy (usually in low dose) should be substituted for sodium cromoglycate if breakthrough symptoms occur or if sodium cromoglycate fails to achieve good control of the symptoms and signs of asthma within 6 weeks (**Fig. 15.1**). Such a switch to

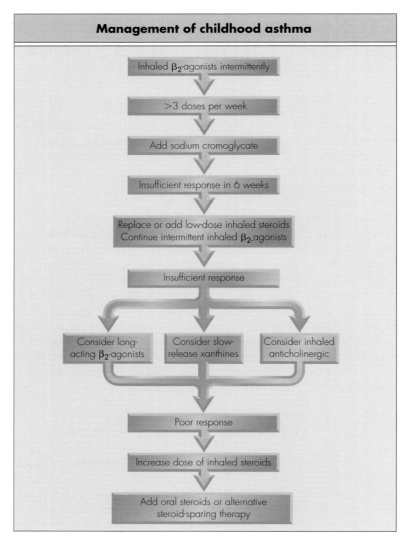

Management of childhood asthma

Inhaled β₂-agonists intermittently

>3 doses per week

Add sodium cromoglycate

Insufficient response in 6 weeks

Replace or add low-dose inhaled steroids
Continue intermittent inhaled β₂-agonists

Insufficient response

Consider long-acting β₂-agonists

Consider slow-release xanthines

Consider inhaled anticholinergic

Poor response

Increase dose of inhaled steroids

Add oral steroids or alternative steroid-sparing therapy

Fig. 15.1. A therapeutic algorithm for the management of childhood asthma. This was prepared by an International Paediatric Asthma Consensus Group and it demonstrates the progression from the management of mild asthma, treated with inhaled β₂-agonists alone, through moderate asthma, treated initially with sodium cromoglycate, to severe asthma treated with inhaled steroids, which may sometimes need to be supplemented by the use of long-acting bronchodilators, or by an increase in the dose of inhaled steroid. (Modified from: Warner *et al., Arch Dis Child* 1992;**67**:240–8.)

inhaled steroid therapy is often required in children with frequent episodic asthma. Trials are currently in progress to assess the relative value of inhaled steroids and cromones (sodium cromoglycate or nedocromil) as first-line therapy in this group of patients.

CHRONIC PERENNIAL AND SEVERE ASTHMA

Children with severe asthma usually do not respond to sodium cromoglycate. They require treatment with potent, topically active inhaled steroid preparations, such as beclomethasone dipropionate (BDP), budesonide or fluticasone. The use of inhaled steroids has dramatically improved the management of severe asthma.

In therapeutic doses, inhaled steroids have only a very low systemic activity, with minimal effects on adrenal function. In very low doses, they have no detectable effect on short-term or long-term growth. Larger doses have been shown to have subtle effects on short-term growth, assessed by knemometry, and, in some studies, also on long-term growth. Severe asthma itself affects growth; and children with severe asthma often receive repeated courses of oral steroid therapy. These factors, together with the sporadic nature of normal growth, tend to confound attempts to investigate the effects of inhaled steroids on growth in childhood. If inhaled steroids have potential growth-retarding effects, however, these are likely to be significantly less than those of the dose of oral steroid which would be necessary to achieve an equivalent degree of asthma control.

The dose of inhaled steroid should be adjusted, depending on progress, and the minimum dose required to control the patient's asthma should be sought.

The lung deposition of inhaled steroid is strongly influenced by the inhaler device through which the drug is administered (*see* Chapter 10). In general, a pMDI used with a spacer device achieves a higher deposition than a pMDI used alone. Dry powder inhalers differ in their performance. For example, budesonide Turbuhaler achieves a greater lung deposition than budesonide pMDI, but this is not necessarily true of other dry powder inhalers. It is essential to consider the properties of both the drug and the device when establishing or adjusting the dose of inhaled therapy in childhood asthma. A change of device may sometimes prove as effective as a change of dose. The suitability of different inhalation devices depends upon the age and the degree of co-operation of the child (*see* page 93).

Where the dose of inhaled steroid is creeping up, the addition of a long-acting bronchodilator, in the form of oral theophylline, inhaled long-acting β_2-agonist or inhaled anticholinergic may be considered (*see* **Fig. 15.1**).

Occasional patients whose asthma is not controlled by high-dose inhaled steroid may need alternative additional therapy. Traditionally, oral steroid therapy has been introduced at this stage, but other possibilities include:

- Regular nebulised budesonide therapy.
- Continuous subcutaneous β_2-agonist infusions.
- Alternative oral anti-inflammatory therapy (e.g. with methotrexate).

OTHER THERAPY

Many other forms of therapy may be used in childhood asthma (**Fig. 15.2**), but not all of these are helpful (*see also* Chapter 11).

Physical activity is important for all children. Swimming is less likely to induce bronchospasm than other forms of sport (**Fig. 15.3**), but pre-dosing with a β_2-agonist should allow children to participate in all forms of sport and exercise.

Institutional care is very rarely required, although it may still be appropriate where considerable absence from school with severe asthma compromises education.

ACUTE ASTHMA

Acute exacerbations of asthma in childhood can be divided into three categories: mild, moderate and severe.

- Mild episodes are associated with an audible wheeze but no significant distress or disturbance of

Treatment possibilities in childhood asthma, classified according to their value	
Proven value	Allergen avoidance β_2-agonists Oral theophylline Inhaled sodium cromoglycate Inhaled steroids Nebulised steroids Oral steroids
Occasional / possible value	Physiotherapy Psychotherapy Anticholinergics Antihistamines
No value / harmful	Immunotherapy Hypnosis Acupuncture Sedation Antibiotics Mucolytics Cough suppressants

Fig. 15.2. Treatment possibilities in childhood asthma, classified according to their value.

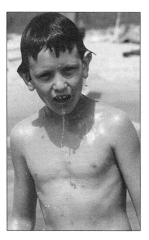

Fig. 15.3. Swimming is less likely to induce bronchospasm than many other forms of exercise. Many children with asthma particularly enjoy swimming for this reason, although pre-dosing with a β_2-agonist should allow participation in most forms of sport. Exercise should be encouraged, because increased physical fitness is often associated with a reduction in the frequency and severity of asthma.

activity and lung function measurements above 70–75% of predicted values. Such episodes may be treated with a low to moderate dose of inhaled β-agonist alone, although this may need to be repeated on a few occasions.

- Moderate acute asthma is associated with a wheeze, the use of accessory muscles, increased respiration rate and some limitation of activity. Lung function is between 50–75% of predicted values. Most children in this category respond to large doses of inhaled β-agonist. However, failure to respond or rapid relapse after a dose would indicate the need for a short course of oral steroids until normal lung function is attained. This may be for as short a period as 1, 2 or 3 days.

- Severe acute asthma is characterised by cyanosis,

severe distress and recession and, in the most severe category, a diminishing wheeze due to diminished air entry to the lungs. Such patients are virtually bed bound and unable to utter more than a word or two between breaths. These children require full high-dependency care with the administration of oxygen, oxygen saturation monitoring, high dose inhaled β-agonist, oral or intravenous steroids and access to intensive care if there is no immediate response. The care of these children follows the same principles as that of adults with acute severe asthma (*see* Chapter 17) and is summarised in **Fig. 15.4**. As in adults, complications of acute severe asthma, including pulmonary lobar collapse (**Fig. 15.5**) and pneumothorax, should be considered if the response to therapy is poor.

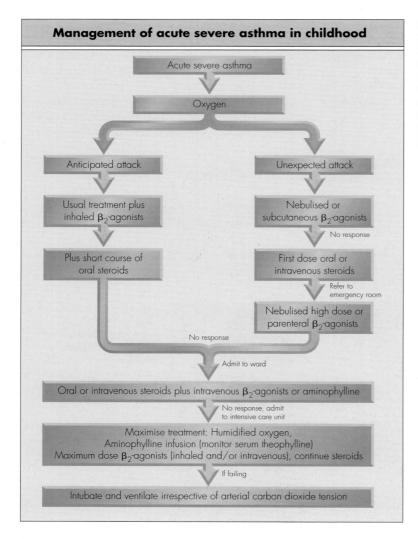

Fig. 15.4. An algorithm for the management of acute severe asthma in childhood. *The suggested management varies for anticipated and unanticipated attacks. Patients should always be admitted to a high-dependency area and intensive care is required if there is evidence of significant oxygen desaturation. (Warner et al., Arch Dis Child 1992;**67**:240–8.)*

An acute attack of asthma always denotes a failure of long-term control. The child's management should be comprehensively reviewed, with special reference to the adequacy of preventive anti-inflammatory therapy and to compliance with prescribed therapy.

INHALATION DEVICES IN CHILDHOOD ASTHMA

The available inhalation devices for asthma therapy can all deliver many particles in the optimal size range to the lungs (*see* Chapter 10), but their ability to do this is usually dependent upon a degree of co-operation from the user. This poses particular problems in the treatment of children.

The range of commonly available inhalation devices is summarised in **Fig. 15.6**, which also shows which drugs can be delivered by which devices, and which devices are likely to be most suitable for children in different age groups.

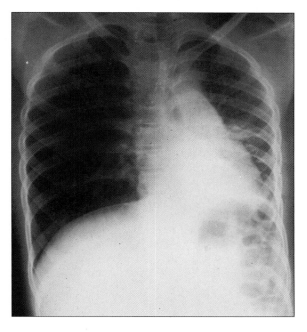

Fig. 15.5. Acute asthma associated with left lower lobe collapse. This child had an acute exacerbation of asthma, with a degree of oxygen desaturation out of proportion to the apparent severity of the attack. The chest radiograph demonstrates the cause of this as left lower lobe collapse. The right lung is over-inflated, with six anterior ends of ribs above the mid-diaphragmatic point. On the left, the hemithorax looks small. The diaphragmatic silhouette is lost and there is a dense triangular area behind the heart indicative of left lower lobe collapse. Shunting of blood through the collapsed lung produced severe hypoxia.

Inhalation devices in the treatment of childhood asthma			
Age (years)	Inhalation device	Relieving treatment	Preventive treatment
<2	Nebuliser and air compressor or valved spacer and face mask	Salbutamol Terbutaline Ipratropium bromide	Sodium cromoglycate Budesonide
2–4	Metered dose inhaler with valved spacer: Nebuhaler Volumatic Aerochamber Fisonair Nebuliser for acute episodes	Terbutaline Salbutamol Ipratropium bromide –	Budesonide BDP – Sodium cromoglycate
5–8	Powder inhalers: Spinhaler Diskhaler Rotahaler Diskus/Accuhaler Turbuhaler/Turbohaler Metered dose inhaler with valved spacer for acute attacks instead of nebuliser	– Salbutamol Salbutamol Salmeterol Terbutaline, Salbutamol All of the above	Sodium cromoglycate BDP, Fluticasone BDP – Budesonide High dose inhaled steroids
>8	Autohaler Metered dose inhaler *with training* or powder inhalers	Salbutamol All of the above	Sodium cromoglycate, BDP All of the above

Fig. 15.6. Inhalation devices in the treatment of childhood asthma. The suitability of devices depends upon the age and degree of co-operation of the child. The table also shows which drugs can be administered through which devices. (Modified from: Warner *et al.*, *Arch Dis Child* 1992;**67**:240–248).

In uncooperative subjects, such as those under 18-months-old, only nebulised inhalation therapy is possible and this is usually delivered by jet nebuliser (**Figs 10.24, 15.7, 15.8**), although ultrasonic nebulisers are also suitable for delivering drugs from solution (they are not suitable for use with particulate suspensions such as budesonide). A driving flow of air (or oxygen in acute asthma) at a rate of at least 6 L/min is required for optimal use, and the characteristics of the nebuliser chamber and the driving compressor determine the speed and efficiency of nebulisation. Speed of nebulisation is a particularly important determinant of compliance with therapy in children, and compliance beyond about 10 minutes of nebulising time is very unlikely. Most anti-asthma drugs are available in a nebulisable form (*see*

Fig. 15.6), but the only effectively nebulisable steroid is budesonide.

An alternative method of administration of inhaled therapy to infants is the combination of a pMDI with a spacer device and a face mask (**Fig. 15.9**). Various shapes and sizes of spacer are available for use with different drugs, but the performance characteristics of some spacers are unknown, and most may deliver variable doses of aerosol to the patient (*see* Chapter 10).

Beyond 18-months-of-age and up to school age, it is usually best to administer pressurised aerosols via a valved spacer device with a face mask or, as soon as practicable, with a mouthpiece (**Fig. 15.10**). These devices have several advantages over the use of a simple pMDI. Most importantly, they overcome the

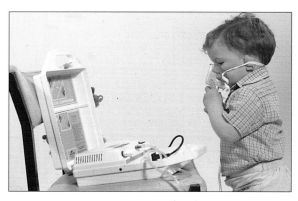

Fig. 15.7. A 2-year-old child using a nebuliser system for his prophylactic asthma medication. The air compressor is on the chair and the nebuliser chamber is in his hand. Most powerful compressors need mains electricity, but foot-pump operated models are also available. This child is using a face mask, but mouthpiece inhalation is preferable whenever possible (as often in older children – see **Fig. 15.8**), as it maximises the inhalation of nebulised aerosol and minimises the risk of local side effects on the face or eyes.

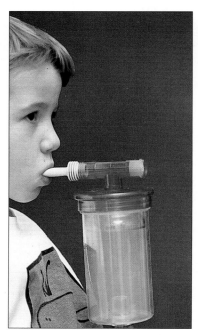

Fig. 15.8. An older child using a nebuliser system with a mouthpiece. The nebuliser chamber is out of the picture. Between it and the mouthpiece is a large reservoir (the 'Mizer' device). This reduces the loss of drug substance into the atmosphere during expiration. The nebuliser output continues throughout the respiratory cycle, but non-inspired mist collects in the reservoir.

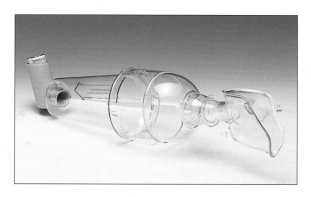

Fig. 15.9. A large volume spacer device fitted with a face mask. The relative portability of the spacer makes administration of medication much simpler to arrange than with a nebuliser. The valve is removed from the spacer device when the face mask is fitted so that the infant simply breathes in and out of the spacer for a short period of time while therapy is administered. Many small and large volume spacer devices are available, but it is important to use a combination of drug, pMDI, spacer and mask which have been designed for compatibility.

need to co-ordinate inhalation with actuation of the inhaler. In addition, they improve delivery to the airways by as much as 50% (*see* Chapter 10). This is particularly important for inhaled steroids, as it increases the delivery of drug to the airway and reduces the total body dose, thus reducing the risk of systemic side-effects.

Above 4-years-of-age, most children can be trained to use any inhalers. The dry powder inhalation devices are generally preferable, at least below the age of 8 years, as less co-ordination is required with these inhalers than with standard pMDIs (*see* Chapter 10). A number of dry powder inhaler devices are available (**Figs 15.11, 15.12**), some of which are pre-loaded with multiple doses. The function of powder inhalers is dependent on an adequate inspiratory force, because the particles must be broken up by the turbulence of inspiratory flow, but even in acute asthma most children can achieve the necessary flow.

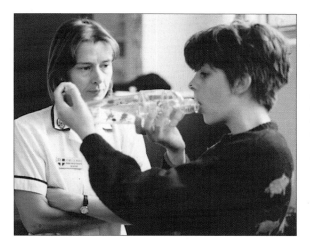

Fig. 15.10. A pMDI fitted with a valved large volume spacer device and a mouthpiece is a valuable method of administration of therapy, especially to children in the age range 2–4 years, and in older children during acute exacerbations of asthma. The device overcomes the problems associated with incoordination between actuation of the pMDI and inhalation, although it is now clear that drug delivery from the spacer may be affected by variable electrostatic charging of its walls (*see* Chapter 10). Here, an older patient is being instructed in the correct use of the Nebuhaler, designed to be used with both budesonide and terbutaline pMDIs.

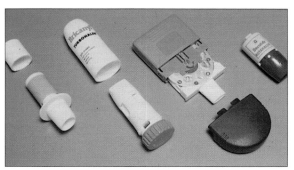

Fig. 15.11. A selection of dry powder inhaler devices which can be used by most children over the age of 5 years. From left to right, these are: the Spinhaler, which must be loaded with an individual capsule of drug before each use; the Turbuhaler (Turbohaler in some countries), which is pre-loaded with 50–200 doses; the Diskhaler, which is loaded with a disc containing eight individual doses; the Rotahaler, which must be loaded with an individual capsule of drug before each use. All these devices have the advantage that the patient's inspiration draws in the dry powder; there is no risk of poor co-ordination between inspiration and drug release.

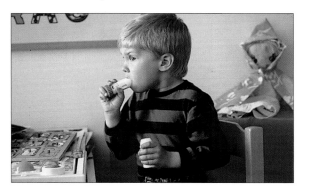

Fig. 15.12. A dry powder inhaler in use. This is a Turbuhaler (Turbohaler), here used to deliver dry powder terbutaline. Most children over the age of 5 years can master the technique of using powder inhalers, and sometimes much younger children can also do so.

Pressurised metered dose inhalers (pMDIs) can be used by many older children (**Fig. 15.13**). Skill and good co-ordination are necessary to optimise the deposition of aerosol in the small airways. The low cost of many pMDIs contributes to their continued widespread use in adolescents and adults.

EDUCATION

All families with asthmatic children require knowledge about the condition and its treatment. Many studies have shown that an improved understanding aids management (*see* Chapter 12). It is essential that children, their parents and their teachers know how to use their prescribed inhalers. The manufacturer usually provides full recommendations with each device, but some key points are summarised in **Fig. 15.14**.

The other key message that must be accepted by families is the difference between the prophylactic (preventive) and relief therapy. Action plans must be agreed between patients, families and doctors, which will give guidance not only on long-term management, but also on appropriate adjustments to therapy as exacerbations occur.

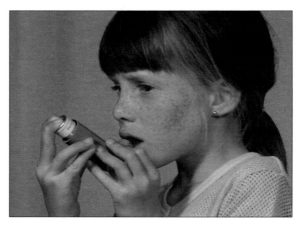

Fig. 15.13. A child about to use a pressurised metered dose inhaler (pMDI). It is essential that children are educated in the correct use of all inhalers, and the need for co-ordination between inspiration and actuation often leads to particular problems for those who use pMDIs. The supervising physician and/or asthma nurse specialist should always observe the child's use of any inhaler device, and arrange further training or the provision of an alternative device if necessary.

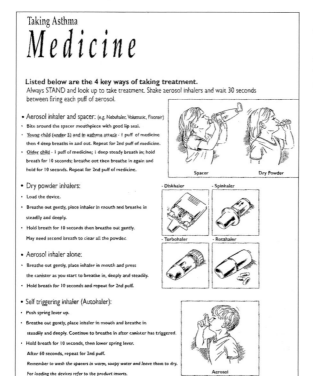

Fig. 15.14. A poster summarising the key points to be observed by a child in using inhaler devices. This was prepared principally for use in schools by the Group for Asthma Management and Education in Southampton Schools (GAMES). It has helped teachers, as well as parents, to ensure that children use inhaled therapy correctly.

16 CHRONIC ASTHMA IN ADULTS

BACKGROUND

The recognition that chronic asthma is an inflammatory disorder has had a major influence on its management. In the past, a patient who had continuing regular or intermittent symptoms but no acute exacerbations was generally considered to have adequately controlled asthma. Patients were often encouraged to tolerate continuing symptoms, treating them when necessary with repeated doses of inhaled β_2-agonist. Such a state would no longer be considered to represent satisfactory control. The underlying inflammatory process in the airways continues in these circumstances and may lead to progressive deterioration in lung function. The term 'good control' now implies the elimination of symptoms and the maintenance of the patient in a normal or near-normal state (*see* page 102).

Until quite recently, bronchodilator agents were regarded as core therapy for all patients, and other agents were usually added only when symptoms reached an unacceptable level of frequency or severity. The therapeutic emphasis has, however, now shifted to agents that suppress the underlying inflammation, and anti-inflammatory drugs—especially inhaled steroids—are now recognised as the most important component of therapy in most patients.

Bronchodilator agents, especially inhaled β_2-agonists, still have an important role in the management of asthma as treatment for patients with mild, episodic symptoms, and as 'relief' therapy in patients with more severe asthma. The routine treatment of chronic asthma with regular bronchodilator therapy alone is, however, now avoided, as it does not deal with the underlying inflammation and may leave the patient at risk of unpredictable acute exacerbations. Such exacerbations require increases in therapy—usually an increased dose of bronchodilator combined with a course of systemic steroid therapy (*see* Chapter 17)—and they often necessitate emergency room attendance or hospital admission. Exacerbations are always unpleasant for the patient, and they are dangerous—most deaths from asthma occur during acute exacerbations. Exacerbations are also the greatest economic burden in the management of asthma, as acute severe asthma accounts for up to 60% of the direct costs of asthma treatment.

Regular bronchodilator therapy has been shown to be associated with an increase in bronchial reactivity. Some studies have also linked regular or excessive β_2-agonist treatment with increased mortality in asthma, although this remains a contentious issue (*see* page 11).

The current aims of asthma management include near-complete control, with the elimination of symptoms, the maintenance of the patient in a normal or near-normal state and the prevention of exacerbations (**Fig. 16.1**). This level of control can usually be achieved by treatment with regular inhaled steroid therapy, and this approach has

---

The principal aims of treatment in asthma

- To prevent or minimise symptoms, rather than to treat them as they occur

- To permit normal activities in daily life

- To achieve normal or best possible lung function

- To limit β_2-agonist therapy to symptomatic rather than regular use

- To avoid side effects from therapy

Fig. 16.1. The principal aims of treatment in asthma.

Advantages of inhaled steroid therapy in asthma

- Improved control of asthma symptoms

- Reduction in acute exacerbations

- Prevention or reversal of airway inflammation

- Reduction in airway hyperresponsiveness (AHR)

- Generally well tolerated, with few clinical side effects

- Cost-effective when compared with bronchodilator therapy

Fig. 16.2. Advantages of inhaled steroid therapy in asthma.

several advantages, including the suppression of airway inflammation, reduction of airway hyperresponsiveness (AHR) and reduction in the risk of acute exacerbations (**Fig. 16.2**).

INHALED STEROID THERAPY IN ASTHMA

Biopsy studies in patients with asthma have confirmed the anti-inflammatory effect of regular inhaled steroid therapy. In patients with early asthma, regular inhaled steroid therapy may lead to the complete reversal of airway inflammation (**Figs 16.3, 16.4**).

A further potential benefit of good early control in asthma, with suppression of inflammation, is the prevention of irreversible structural changes in the airway

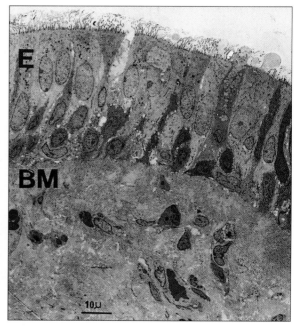

Fig. 16.3. The inflammatory nature of asthma can be confirmed by electron microscopy. This section of the airway wall comes from a patient with asthma of 9 months' duration, who had received only symptomatic treatment with inhaled β_2-agonist alone. The airway epithelium (E) is severely damaged, and an intense inflammatory reaction can be seen beneath the basement membrane (BM). Several types of inflammatory cell can be identified, including eosinophils (Eo), lymphocytes (L) and degranulated mast cells (M). These changes reflect the presence of a chronic inflammatory process in the airway wall (Laitinen *et al.*, *J Allergy Clin Immunol* 1992; **90**: 32–42).

Fig. 16.4. An electron micrograph of a section of the airway wall from the same patient as in Fig.16.3, obtained **3 months later** (asthma duration 12 months), after regular treatment for 3 months with inhaled budesonide, 600 mg b.d. The airway epithelium (E) has been normalised, and no inflammatory changes were seen beneath the basement membrane (BM) (Laitinen *et al.*, *J Allergy Clin Immunol* 1992; **90**: 32–42).

wall. Reversible asthma may progress to fixed irreversible obstruction if inflammatory change is persistent (*see* Chapter 2). Basement membrane thickening is followed by subepithelial fibrosis and smooth muscle hyperplasia and hypertrophy (**Fig. 16.5**), and these changes are associated with progressive deterioration in lung function.

Retrospective studies have shown that the degree of irreversibility in asthma is related to the extent of earlier difficulties in establishing asthma control, and a recent prospective study has shown that the duration of symptoms before the initiation of inhaled steroid therapy has a significant influence on the degree of resulting improvement in lung function: the sooner inhaled steroids are started, the greater the improvement in lung function (**Fig. 16.6**).

A number of studies in adults and children have confirmed that early intervention with inhaled steroids produces better symptom control and reduction in airway reactivity than β_2-agonist therapy used alone. **Figures 16.7** and **16.8** show the results of a recent 2-year study in Finland. In an extension of this study, when a group who had taken β_2-agonist alone for 2 years switched to inhaled steroid they failed to improve to the same extent as those who had taken inhaled steroid from the

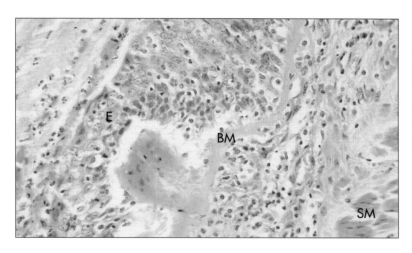

Fig. 16.5. Light microscopy of a large airway in asthma (original magnification, x80). The epithelium (E) is infiltrated with inflammatory cells and is beginning to separate – a prelude to epithelial shedding. There is marked thickening of the basement membrane (BM), with further infiltration and smooth muscle hypertrophy and hyperplasia (SM) below.

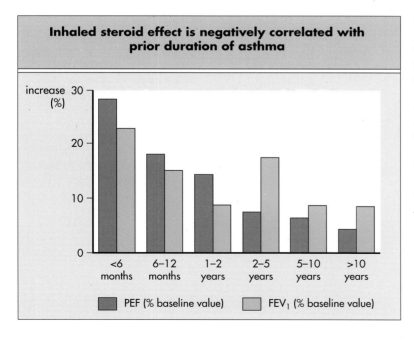

Fig. 16.6. The maximum responses seen in PEF and FEV$_1$, correlated with the duration of asthma prior to the start of inhaled steroid therapy. Values are expressed as percentage increases in the baseline readings in each group of patients. There were strong negative correlations between duration of asthma symptoms at the time of initiation of inhaled budesonide therapy and the degree of improvement in both PEF and FEV$_1$. (Based on data from Selroos *et al.*, *Am J Respir Crit Care Med* 1994; **149** (suppl): A211.)

beginning of the study (**Fig. 16.9**). Indeed, the improvement achieved in the 'late intervention' group after inhaled steroid treatment for 1 year was no greater than that achieved in the 'early intervention' group after 1 week of inhaled steroid treatment.

The group who had been given inhaled steroid for 2 years and then stopped the drug gradually lost the benefit of better control and reduced airway reactivity, even though good control had been maintained throughout the first 2 years (**Fig. 16.9**). Thus inhaled steroid therapy controlled the symptoms, signs and underlying mechanisms of asthma in these patients but did not 'cure' the condition, a finding that is consistent with that of other studies.

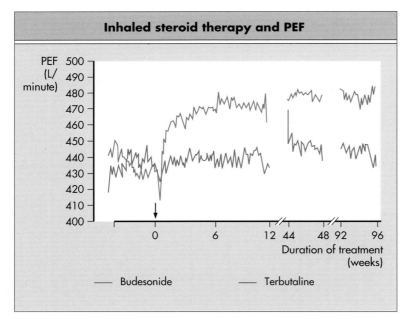

Fig. 16.7. Morning PEF in the two groups of patients in the Finnish multicentre study of early intervention with inhaled steroid therapy (budesonide) in patients with newly diagnosed asthma (pre-treatment duration up to 12 months). The significant difference between the steroid-treated patients and those treated with inhaled β_2-agonist (terbutaline) alone persisted throughout the study period (Haahtela *et al.*, *N Engl J Med* 1991; **325**; 388–92).

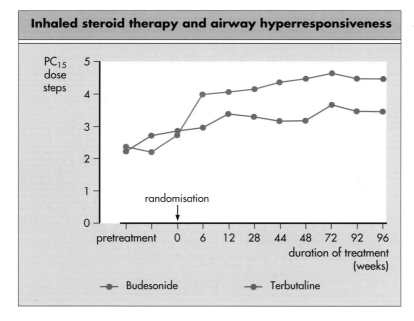

Fig. 16.8. Airway hyperresponsiveness as assessed by PC_{15} histamine dose steps in the two groups of patients in the Finnish multicentre early intervention study. The lesser degree of airway reactivity in the steroid-treated patients developed within 6 weeks and persisted throughout the study period (Haahtela *et al.*, *N Engl J Med* 1991; **325**; 388–92).

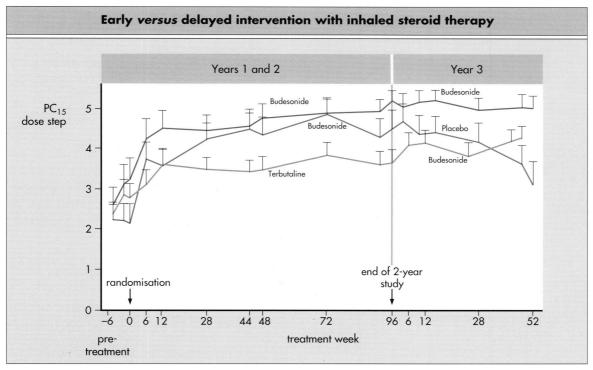

Fig. 16.9. Airway hyperresponsiveness as assessed by PC_{15} histamine dose steps in the first and second phases of the Finnish multicentre early intervention study. The results for the group treated with steroids in the first phase, shown as one group in **Figs 16.7** and **16.8**, have here been divided in both phases, according to the treatment they received in phase 2. Inhaled steroid (budesonide) treatment led to improved airway reactivity in both groups in phase 1. This improvement was maintained by a lower dose of inhaled steroid but worsened by the substitution of placebo in phase 2. Patients treated with inhaled steroid after a delay of two years also improved, but not to the same degree as those who were treated with inhaled steroid from the start of the study (Haahtela *et al.*, *N Engl J Med*, 1994; **331**: 700–5).

STEPPED CARE IN ASTHMA

Traditionally, the management of asthma has followed the 'step-up' approach. Initial small doses of therapy are progressively increased at intervals, and additional drugs may be added (or substituted) and increased in a similar way, until the condition is brought under good control. Once good control is achieved and maintained, attempts may be made to return down the steps and reduce the dose of therapy, so that the minimum possible long-term maintenance dose is used (**Fig. 16.10**).

There is increasing interest in an alternative to the 'step-up' approach, which may prove to be appropriate for the control of asthma with inhaled steroid therapy in some or all patients. This is a 'step-down' approach, in which higher doses of therapy are used initially, with the aim of bringing the condition under full control as rapidly as possible. The initial higher dose therapy is usually a course of oral steroids or high dose inhaled steroids. As in the 'step-up' approach, once good control is achieved and maintained, attempts can be made to reduce the dose of therapy, so that the minimum possible long-term maintenance dose is used (**Fig. 16.11**).

Currently published guidelines for the management of asthma follow the 'step-up' approach, but the 'step-down' approach may be more rational if the aim is to suppress inflammation rapidly and prevent the development of irreversible changes in the airways. Some current research is focused on the 'step-down' approach, and it is often used in practice by many asthma specialists.

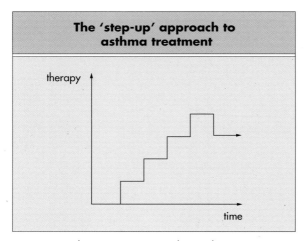

Fig. 16.10. The 'step-up' approach to asthma treatment.

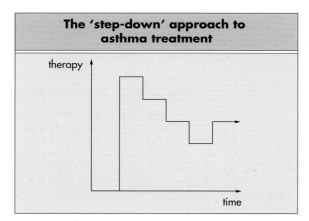

Fig. 16.11. The 'step-down' approach to asthma treatment.

CONTROL IN ASTHMA

Ideal control of asthma is the absence of any symptoms with no treatment and no restriction of lifestyle. This can be achieved only by identification of specific triggers that can be avoided easily. In practice this is unusual.

Good control is the presence of minimal or no symptoms with no acute exacerbations and minimal or no adverse effects of therapy and no restriction of activities. Control can be assessed on subjective criteria such as symptoms and on objective criteria such as peak flow variability. Circadian variation of less than 20% with mean peak flow >80% of predicted or best achievable would indicate good control (**Figs 16.12, 16.13**). Criteria that can be used to define good control are:

- Minimal (ideally no) chronic symptoms.
- No nocturnal symptoms.
- No acute exacerbations.
- Minimal need for short-acting bronchodilators.
- No limitation of activity, including exercise.
- Circadian variability of peak flow <20%.
- Peak flow >80% predicted or best achievable.
- Minimal (ideally no) adverse effects from treatment.

For patients further into a stepped care treatment programme such a level of control may not be achievable; the least possible symptoms, bronchodilator use, peak flow variability and adverse effects of treatment would be the aims of management.

GUIDELINES FOR ASTHMA MANAGEMENT

Audits of asthma care have demonstrated problems in the management of both acute and chronic asthma. In an attempt to improve the general standard of care of patients with asthma various sets of guidelines have been developed and published at national and international levels (**Fig. 16.14**). The British Thoracic Society collaborated with a number of other agencies to produce a stepped care version in 1990. This was updated in a revised set of guidelines in 1993, with collaboration from paediatric, accident and emergency and general practitioner groups. The guidelines outlined in this chapter are based broadly on those published by the British Thoracic Society in 1993, but have been influenced by other published guidelines and by developments since that date.

Guidelines provide an outline of appropriate care for correctly diagnosed patients, but it is essential that each patient should be individually assessed and managed. Communication and education, which are vital to compliance and to patient care, are part of the individual doctor–patient relationship and cannot always follow a pre-defined formula.

There is a risk that guidelines might limit research or lag behind new developments in asthma management. Used properly, they can help to identify areas of uncertainty to which clinical research should be directed, but they must be supplemented or updated regularly to incorporate possible changes in management (such as the 'step-down' approach).

Successful care of asthma requires an integrated approach aimed at forming a partnership between patient, family and doctor. This may need to be

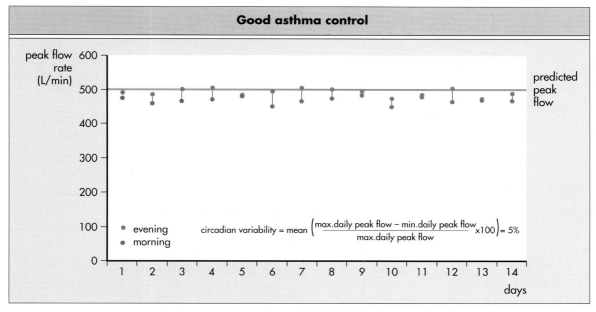

Fig. 16.12. Good asthma control. Most evening peak flows are as predicted, with daily variability of only 5%.

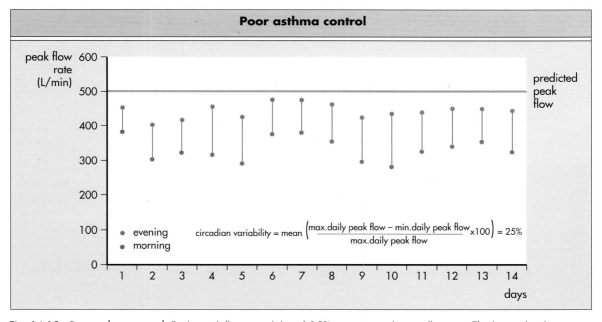

Fig. 16.13. Poor asthma control. Daily peak flow variability of 25% mean, i.e. abnormally great. The lowest levels occur in the morning.

developed over time. Patients will not remember all the necessary information from one consultation and back-up in the form of written and visual material is likely to be helpful (*see* Chapter 12). Written material is more successful if it can be made personal for each patient. Notes and diagrams produced with the patient during the consultation can be most useful in this process of collaboration (**Fig. 16.15**). At first this may be information on inhaler use and peak flow monitoring, but the aim should be to develop a self-management plan, allowing control of asthma with adjustments in treatment by the patient according to regular monitoring of symptoms and peak flow records.

In line with current 'step-up' guidelines, the management of chronic asthma may be divided into a preliminary step, followed by five further steps of increasing therapy (**Fig. 16.16**). Some general considerations apply to all steps of asthma management (**Fig. 16.17**).

Some published guidelines for the management of asthma		
Country	Date	Reference
Australia and New Zealand	1989	Med J Australia **151**: 650–3
UK	1990 1993	BMJ **301**: 651–3 Thorax **48** (suppl.): S1–S24
Canada	1990	J Allergy Clin Immunol **85**: 1098–111
USA	1991	J Allergy Clin Immunol **88**: 425–534
Sweden	1992	Läkartidningen **89**: 2608–11
International	1992	Clin Exp Allergy **22** (Suppl.): S1–S72
International – Paediatric	1992	Arch Dis Child **67**: 240–8
World Health Organization	–	In preparation

Fig. 16.14. Some published guidelines for the management of asthma.

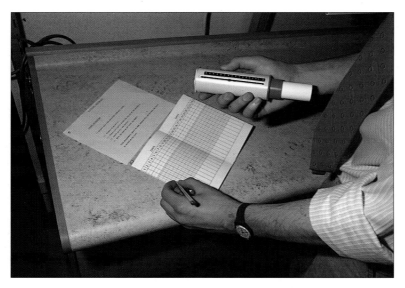

Fig. 16.15. Notes and diagrams produced with the patient during the consultation can be a valuable part of the process of collaboration between prescriber and patient.

Fig. 16.16. The step care of patients with chronic asthma.

The stepped care of patients with chronic asthma

Preliminary step

Identify provoking factors
• Reduce when possible

Step 1

Occasional inhaled short-acting ß$_2$-agonist
• Go to Step 2 if used more often than once per day/three times per week

Step 2

Regular anti-inflammatory agent
• Usually inhaled steroid up to 800 µg/day

Step 3

Moderate to high dose inhaled steroid – 1000–2000 µg/day
• Via large volume spacer
• Or dry powder with mouth rinsing
Or continue as Step 2 but add:
• Long-acting inhaled bronchodilator
• Long-acting oral bronchodilator
• Nedocromil sodium

Step 4

Moderate to high dose inhaled steroid – 1000–2000 µg/day
• Via large volume spacer
• Or dry powder with mouth rinsing
And add:
• Long-acting inhaled bronchodilator
• Long-acting oral bronchodilator
• Consider nebulised steroid

Step 5

Add oral steroid therapy

General considerations in the management of chronic asthma at all steps of treatment

- Aim for control which permits the patient's desired lifestyle, rather than modifying that lifestyle

- Monitor control by PEF measurement in clinic and (often) by patient

- Teach and check inhaler technique

- Assess patient compliance with prescibed therapy

- Review treatment regularly

- Establish criteria for initiation of short-course oral steroid therapy (initiated by patient when suitably educated and experienced)

- Attempt step down of therapy at any stage after period of stability

Fig. 16.17. General considerations in the management of chronic asthma at all steps of treatment.

Preliminary step

Identify provoking factors
- Reduce when possible

The preliminary step is to identify any precipitating causes (triggers) for asthma and to seek to eliminate them. These may include:
- **Drugs**. β-blockers as tablets or even eye drops, aspirin and non-steroidal anti-inflammatory drugs.
- **Smoking**. Active and passive.
- **Occupational exposure**. This may need careful enquiry and peak flow monitoring.
- **Airborne allergens**. Pets, pollens, house dust mite: avoid if possible or consider ways to reduce exposure.
- **Exercise, cold air**. These should be managed by adjustments in treatment rather than avoidance.

Most patients with asthma have multiple sensitivities and cannot resolve all their problems by simple avoidance measures. However, in some cases this may be possible, particularly with drug-induced asthma, occupational asthma (**Fig. 16.18**) or animal exposure (**Fig. 16.19**). The opportunities for prevention should be considered carefully in every case. Even when there are multiple provoking agents, limitation of exposure to some factors may improve control or limit the extent of drug therapy. Exposure to an allergen has been shown to worsen control and increase responsiveness to other triggers for several days.

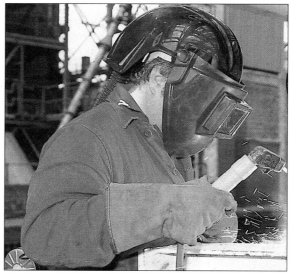

Fig. 16.18. Avoidance measures may prevent or relieve occupational asthma. Welding can be associated with a number of lung problems, including occupational asthma. The particular risks are determined by the composition of the electrodes, the metal and its coating, the flux and any shielding gas.

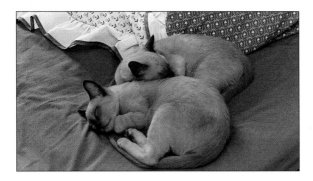

Fig. 16.19. Allergy to cats is common. Cats and other animals should always be banished from bedrooms, and cat-sensitive asthma is an indication for complete removal of cats from the patient's home.

Step 1

Occasional inhaled short-acting β_2-agonist
• Go to Step 2 if used more often than once per day/three times per week

---

Step 1 in therapy is the occasional use of bronchodilators in response to intermittent symptoms. Inhaled selective β_2-receptor agonists are the relief bronchodilator treatment of choice in mild asthma. They should be used as required for asthma symptoms: wheeze, shortness of breath and cough. Many inhaler devices are available (*see* Chapter 10) and almost all patients can be taught to use one of these devices efficiently. Teaching the technique and checking the patient's ability are part of the responsibility of the prescriber (**Fig. 16.20**).

This step may also include the prophylactic use of β_2-agonists before exercise in patients with exercise-induced asthma (*see* page 18).

As mentioned above there is concern that the regular use of β_2-agonists in asthma may worsen control and increase airway reactivity, so the frequency of their use should be monitored by the patient and the prescriber. All published guidelines agree that the patient should progress to Step 2 if a dose of inhaled bronchodilator is needed more frequently than once per day. Some guidelines are more stringent than this, suggesting that the patient should progress to Step 2 if a dose of inhaled bronchodilator is needed more frequently than three times per week.

The key message is that inhaled β_2-agonists alone are no longer considered appropriate therapy for chronic asthma with regular symptoms. Their use as monotherapy should be limited to patients with occasional mild symptoms. Patients with more severe symptoms should be treated at Step 2 or above, although intermittent inhaled β_2-agonists may continue to be used as 'relief' or 'rescue' therapy for symptoms at the higher steps. Indeed, their frequent use at these higher stages is an indication of inadequate underlying control and of the need for a further progression in preventive therapy. Inhaled β_2-agonists should be taken regularly only when there are persistent uncontrolled symptoms despite the maximisation of other appropriate therapy (some patients at Step 4).

Adverse effects of β_2-agonists, such as tremor and palpitations, are occasionally troublesome, but their presence at Step 1 usually indicates excessive use, and the need for a progression to Step 2 with a resulting reduction in β_2-agonist dose.

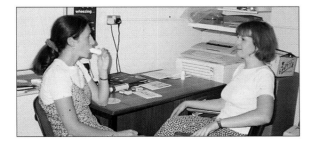

Fig. 16.20. Teaching and checking inhaler technique is an integral part of the prescription of inhaled therapy.

Step 2

Regular anti-inflammatory agent
• Usually inhaled steroid up to 800 µg/day

The next step up from occasional use of bronchodilators is the introduction of inhaled anti-inflammatory agents. The usual agents are inhaled steroids. Alternatives are sodium cromoglycate and nedocromil sodium, but these agents have not been shown to have clinically significant anti-inflammatory effects, and they are now not commonly used in adult patients. A reasonable trial of sodium cromoglycate or nedocromil sodium involves at least 2 months of treatment, and many patients will require further therapy for symptoms during this period. There is some evidence from *in vitro* and *in vivo* studies that theophyllines may also have some anti-inflammatory effects, but the limited clinical evidence means that they cannot be regarded as alternative anti-inflammatory agents at this stage.

The usual starting dose of inhaled corticosteroids in adults is 400–800 µg/day in two doses, but the dose depends on the severity of the asthma and the drug and device prescribed. Different inhaled steroids and different delivery systems are not equipotent (**Fig. 16.21**), so it is always important to specify:
• The drug.
• The dose.
• The delivery device or system.

For example, some dry powder devices, such as the Turbuhaler (Turbohaler), achieve a lung deposition twice as high as that achieved by the same nominal dose from a conventional pressurised metered dose inhaler (*see* Chapter 10).

It may be helpful to use a higher inhaled steroid dose initially to gain asthma control with subsequent reduction to a lower maintenance dose (the 'step-down' approach).

If sodium cromoglycate or nedocromil sodium is used as first therapy but fails to achieve control, then inhaled steroids should be substituted or added. If steroids are used as the first anti-inflammatory agent and control is inadequate with 800 µg daily, then therapy should move to Step 3.

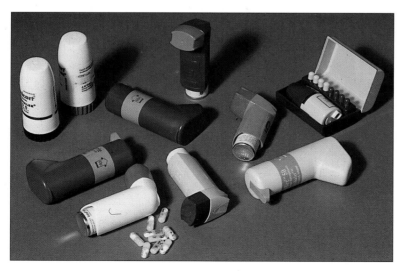

Fig. 16.21. Different inhaled steroids and different delivery devices are not equipotent. In any consideration of therapy it is essential to specify the drug, the dose and the delivery device.

Step 3	
Moderate to high dose inhaled steroid – 1000–2000 µg/day • Via large volume spacer • Or dry powder with mouth rinsing	Or continue as Step 2 but add: • Long-acting inhaled bronchodilator • Long-acting oral bronchodilator • Nedocromil sodium

There are two main strategies at this stage, after low dose steroids fail to produce satisfactory control. Either the dose of inhaled steroids can be increased to 1000–2000 µg daily (a 'moderate' to 'high' dose) or a long-acting bronchodilator can be added to the treatment. The choices of long-acting bronchodilators are inhaled β_2-agonists such as salmeterol or formoterol, oral β_2-agonists such as bambuterol, and oral slow-release theophyllines. The addition of nedocromil sodium to moderate-dose inhaled steroids may be a helpful alternative strategy. Such changes in treatment should be assessed by subjective and objective monitoring. In all these treatment protocols the short-acting inhaled β_2-agonists should continue to be available for use as 'rescue' medication when necessary.

When inhaled steroids are used in doses of over 800 µg pressurised metered dose inhalers should be used with a spacer device to reduce oral deposition (**Fig. 16.22**; *see also* Chapter 10) and the mouth should be rinsed after dry powder inhalation (**Fig. 16.23**). These manoeuvres reduce the amount of swallowed drug and thus limit the risk of systemic absorption from the gut (but not, of course, from the lungs – *see* **Fig 9.5**).

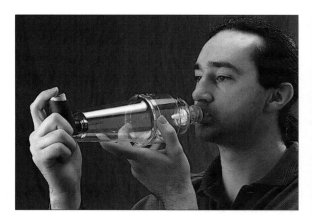

Fig. 16.22. A large volume spacer device increases the lung deposition and reduces the oral deposition of drugs delivered from pMDIs. The reduction of oral deposition is important when prescribing moderate to high doses of inhaled steroid, as this minimises the proportion of each dose which can become systemically available via the gastrointestinal tract.

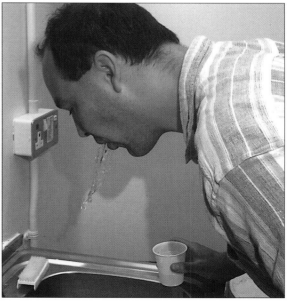

Fig. 16.23. Mouth rinsing can reduce the systemically absorbed portion of each dose from dry powder inhalers. The mouth should be rinsed with water immediately after each dose, and the rinsing water must be discarded. (Patients may swallow the water unless they are specifically told not to.)

Step 4	
Moderate to high dose inhaled steroid – 1000–2000 µg/day • Via large volume spacer • Or dry powder with mouth rinsing	And add: • Long-acting inhaled bronchodilator • Long-acting oral bronchodilator • Consider nebulised steroid

Step 4 involves the combination of more than one of the options from Step 3. The inhaled corticosteroid dose is maintained at or increased to a level of 1000–2000 µg/day, and regular bronchodilator therapy is given using a long-acting oral β_2-agonist, slow-release theophylline or, possibly, an inhaled anticholinergic agent. Conventional short-acting inhaled β_2-agonists are continued as 'rescue' medication when necessary for symptomatic relief.

In patients whose asthma is difficult to control a short course of oral steroids may help to establish control, which can then be maintained with conventional inhaled therapy.

An alternative at this stage may be the use of a nebulised steroid (budesonide is the only steroid currently available for nebulisation), which may help to establish good control without the risk of the need for prolonged or repeated oral steroid therapy, and thus reduce the risk of adverse systemic effects (**Fig. 16.24**). When patients are stepping down from Step 5 to Step 4, nebulised steroids may act as an intermediate stage between systemic and conventional inhaled therapy.

Occasionally it may also be necessary to consider the use of a nebuliser to deliver high doses of inhaled bronchodilators. Nebulised bronchodilators should, however, be authorised as part of home therapy only if the patient and the family are quite clear on the indications for their use and for obtaining further help, so that they do not delay seeking aid during an acute episode.

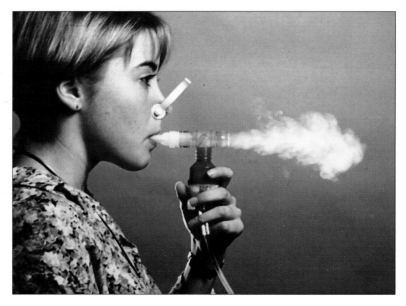

Fig. 16.24. Nebulised therapy may be helpful in severe asthma. High doses of bronchodilators may be delivered by this method in carefully defined circumstances. Nebulised steroid therapy may provide an alternative to oral steroid therapy, or an aid to oral dose reduction.

Step 5

Add oral steroid therapy

The final step in the therapeutic pathway is the addition of regular oral steroids to the therapy specified in Step 4. This is an undesirable option with many side effects (**Figs 16.25–16.27**; *see also* page 52). It should be embarked upon only when compliance and inhalation technique have been fully explored, and after other means of control have failed, including a short course of oral steroids in reducing dosage or possibly a trial of nebulised steroid. Inhaled steroids should be continued with the oral agent to minimise the oral dose.

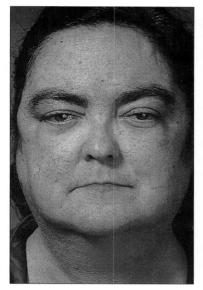

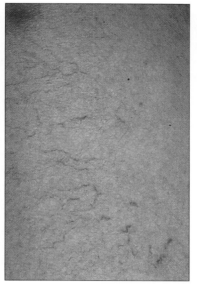

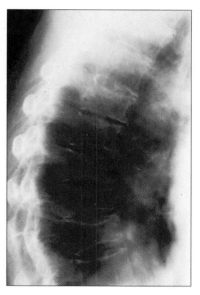

Fig. 16.25. **Cushingoid facial features** resulting from long-term oral steroid therapy for asthma. This 49-year-old woman had received oral steroids over most of the past 20 years, as inhaled steroids had repeatedly failed to control her asthma. In addition to the facial features, she had generally thin skin with striae, frequent episodes of purpura and bruising, and kyphosis associated with osteoporotic vertebral collapse. Fortunately, such extreme cases are rare, but systemic side-effects are an inevitable consequence of prolonged oral steroid therapy. By contrast, they are extremely unusual with inhaled steroid therapy.

Fig. 16.26. **Skin atrophy in a patient with asthma who had been treated with long-term oral steroid therapy.** The patient's thin skin reveals cutaneous blood vessels. It is easily injured, with bruising and bleeding, and heals very slowly. Lesser skin changes of this type have been reported in a few patients receiving long-term high-dose inhaled steroid therapy, but they are extremely rare in these circumstances. The risk of such systemic effects with inhaled therapy can be minimised by using spacer devices or mouth-rinsing, and by selecting steroids with a high first-pass metabolism, such as budesonide and fluticasone, for high-dose inhaled therapy.

Fig. 16.27. **Osteoporosis leading to vertebral collapse in a patient with asthma who had received long-term oral steroid therapy.** This radiograph shows severe osteoporosis with early wedging of vertebral bodies in the mid-thoracic region. Episodes of vertebral collapse are painful, and result in progressive kyphosis. Osteoporosis also makes the patient more susceptible to fractures at the hip, wrist and elsewhere.

Other steps

In severe persistent asthma where continuous oral steroids cannot be avoided, some other approaches may limit the dose of steroids and thus their potential for systemic effects:

- **Addition or progressive substitution of nebulised steroid therapy** (see Step 4 above).

- **Continuous subcutaneous infusion of a β_2-agonist**. This method may help in patients with brittle asthma who deteriorate suddenly or in those with resistant morning dips of peak flow. High tissue levels of β_2-agonist are obtained by this method. The subcutaneous site is changed by the patient every 2–3 days.

- **Methotrexate**. Weekly oral doses of methotrexate may allow reduction of the oral steroid dose over several months. The side effects of methotrexate include bone marrow suppression, liver toxicity and pulmonary fibrosis. The blood picture and liver function tests must be monitored during therapy.

- **Cyclosporin A**. Cyclosporin A has shown benefit in some trials. Blood levels can be measured and the main toxic effects are on the kidney.

Stepping down

The treatment of asthma should be reviewed regularly for each patient.

When asthma is well controlled stepping down of therapy should be considered. When treatment up to Step 4 or 5 has been necessary to establish control this may often be reduced after a short time. On the lower steps, once anti-inflammatory treatment has been started it should be continued to maintain good control of asthma for six months or more before it is reduced or stopped. The patient should then be observed carefully for a return of symptoms, and therapy should be stepped back up if necessary.

Although some patients may enter a state of apparent remission despite the withdrawal of anti-inflammatory therapy with inhaled steroids, they should always be considered to be at risk of further severe asthma. There is evidence that regular anti-inflammatory therapy may prevent permanent damage to the airways, but little evidence that even this apparently successful therapy is truly curative. Many patients may need long-term therapy with anti-inflammatory agents to maintain complete control of asthma, but this can often be continued in relatively low doses.

SPECIAL SITUATIONS

This chapter has reviewed the recommended management for typical adult patients with chronic asthma, but management in some patients is complicated by other factors.

The management of asthma in childhood is discussed in Chapter 15.

The management of a number of other special groups of patients is influenced by other factors, including:
- Exercise-induced asthma.
- Olympic or other sporting regulations.
- Nocturnal asthma.
- Aspirin-induced asthma.
- Pregnancy.

These groups of patients are discussed in Chapter 18.

17 ACUTE SEVERE ASTHMA

INTRODUCTION

Asthma remains a potentially fatal condition despite the great improvement in its treatment over the past 20 years (*see* Chapter 1). There is a persistent mortality from asthma, with deaths occurring at home, during transfer to hospital and in hospital. (20% of asthma deaths in the UK occur after arrival at hospital.)

Acute severe asthma is a life-threatening episode of asthma where the patient is distressed by severe breathlessness with tightness of the chest, and often inability to complete a sentence. The patient may sit with hunched shoulders, leaning forward (**Fig. 17.1**). Confusion and drowsiness are rare, and are associated with hypoxaemia and probable hypercapnia and respiratory acidosis, all suggesting impending death.

Rapid clinical assessment of severity is important, as inadequate assessment by the physician is associated with undertreatment and, possibly, mortality. The main features of a simple assessment, including exercise tolerance, are shown in **Fig. 17.2**. The heart rate is rapid, with possible variation in the pulse strength with respiration (pulsus paradoxus), although absence of this

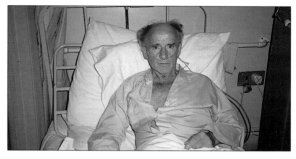

Fig. 17.1. A patient admitted with acute severe asthma. The patient was clearly distressed by breathlessness and is already being treated with oxygen and inhaled therapy. The patient often sits with shoulder muscles braced and leans forward in an attempt to improve breathing.

Assessment of severity of asthma		
Assessment of severity and signs	Scoring system	
	0	1
Loss of exercise tolerance	Able to walk and talk	Unable to walk short distances or complete long sentences
Using accessory muscles, tracheal tug and intercostal recession	Absent	Present
Wheezing	Absent	Present
Respiratory rate (min^{-1})	≤25 (adult) ≤30 (child)	>25 >30
Pulse rate (min^{-1})	≤110 (adult) ≤120 (child)	>110 >120
Palpable pulsus paradoxus	Absent	Present
Peak expiratory flow rate (L/min)	≥100	<100

Fig. 17.2. Assessment of severity of asthma. A system for scoring the severity of an attack of acute severe asthma. A total score of 4 or more suggests severe asthma requiring urgent treatment. This assessment can be carried out in less than 2 minutes and does not prevent the initiation of treatment. Cyanosis occurs very late in an attack and, as it suggests imminent death, it has been deliberately omitted from this assessment.

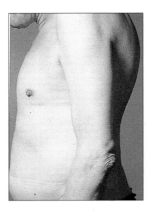

Fig. 17.3. Acute asthma with intercostal recession and hyperinflation. Examination of the patient with acute severe asthma reveals intercostal recession and tracheal tugging during inspiration with marked hyperinflation and a vertical respiratory movement, the chest wall being lifted by the accessory muscles of respiration.

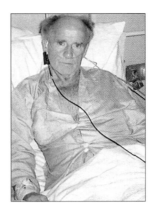

Fig. 17.4. Oxygen saturation measured by pulse oximetry. The introduction of simple, accurate and comparatively cheap devices for measuring oxygen saturation, placing a probe over the finger or ear lobe, has simplified oxygen assessment in asthmatic patients. Severe hypoxaemia can be identified and corrected by increasing the inspired oxygen concentration.

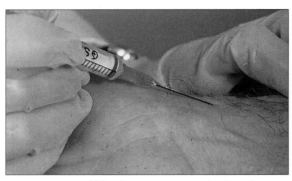

Fig. 17.5. Arterial blood gas estimation. Blood is taken from the radial artery in a patient with severe asthma. This is best taken from the non-dominant hand, after ensuring there is a good ulnar artery flow and injecting a small dose of local anaesthetic.

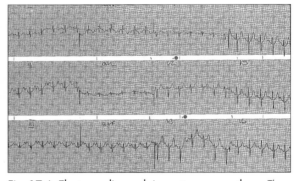

Fig. 17.6. Electrocardiograph in acute severe asthma. The ECG in asthma usually shows tachycardia and may show ischaemia in the elderly. There are frequently changes in amplitude associated with respiration and the heart rate. Following 2 days of intense treatment with oxygen, high-dose inhaled bronchodilators and systemic steroids, this patient's ECG returned to normal.

sign does not exclude severe asthma. Assessment also includes the use of accessory muscles, intercostal recession (**Fig. 17.3**), and the presence of wheeze, all which are simply observed. Wheeze, however, may be absent when asthma is at its most severe.

Measurement of PEF on initial assessment is important, and can be rapidly performed. FEV_1 and PEF can be measured in the home, primary care centre, ambulance or emergency department.

The introduction of pulse oximetry, a simple and non-invasive method of measuring arterial oxygen saturation, has meant the response to increased inspired oxygen can be observed during transfer by ambulance or in the accident and emergency department (**Figs 7.2, 17.4**). Arterial blood gas measurements can be reserved for patients with a low oxygen saturation (< 93%) and for the confused or drowsy patient (**Fig. 17.5**) to determine the presence of hypercapnia and/or respiratory acidosis.

Other investigations at the hospital include plasma electrolyte estimations, particularly potassium, as hypokalaemia may be associated with hyperventilation, β-agonist administration and the metabolic alteration associated with steroid therapy. An ECG may give an indication of right heart strain (**Figs 17.6, 17.7**) and a chest radiograph should be done if there is any doubt as to the presence of a pneumothorax or localised infection.

TREATMENT

The management of acute severe asthma has been the focus of a number of national and international working parties and guidelines have been produced in many countries. The guidelines differ in detail, but the major recommendations are similar throughout the world. The management of acute severe asthma outside hospital is summarised in **Fig. 17.8** and the hospital management is summarised in **Fig. 17.9**. The management of acute severe asthma in childhood is summarised in **Fig. 15.4**. The principles of management are similar in all situations.

Patients with severe acute asthma are terrified and feel they are going to die. Extensive history taking and examination are unnecessary when patients are already taking specific treatment for asthma. Acute severe asthma in most adult patients develops over a few days, so many patients are dehydrated by the time they arrive in hospital, due to the combination of inability to drink and excessive insensible fluid loss from tachypnoea. Fluid replacement may be required and, even if this is unnecessary, intravenous access is a useful general measure during transfer by paramedic ambulance and on arrival at the emergency department.

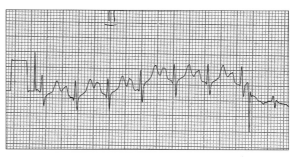

Fig. 17.7. Electrocardiograph in acute severe asthma. During acute severe asthma, severe hypoxia may be associated with the development of acute pulmonary hypertension, when it is identified by the development of an acute 'P' on ECG, most obvious in lead 2 as shown here. Following intensive treatment the abnormal P-waves returned to normal.

Specific treatment

Specific treatment for acute severe asthma at home, in transfer or on arrival at hospital is remarkably similar and consists of oxygen therapy, bronchodilators and steroids. Apart from the administration of oxygen there is no fixed order of treatment, particularly for very ill patients, as all drugs may need to be given simultaneously.

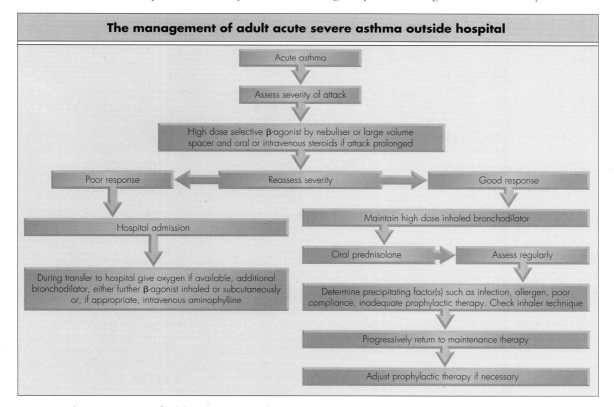

Fig. 17.8. The management of adult acute severe asthma outside hospital.

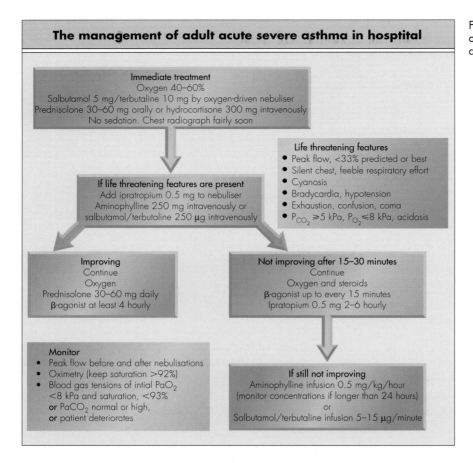

Fig. 17.9. The management of adult acute severe asthma in hospital.

OXYGEN THERAPY

All ill patients with acute severe asthma are hypoxaemic and require oxygen. This should be given via a face mask in a concentration high enough to maintain an adequate arterial oxygen saturation (**Fig 17.10**). The risk of significant carbon dioxide retention is low, particularly in patients who are aged less than 50, and inspired oxygen concentrations of 35–40% should be given rather than the lower 24–28% which is often recommended.

Bronchodilators

β-agonist therapy

Inhaled β-agonist therapy is the first-line therapy. Oxygen driven nebulisers are preferred (**Fig. 17.10**) since β-agonists can potentially worsen hypoxia (rare with inhaled therapy compared with intravenous). An appropriate dose is salbutamol 2.5–5.0 mg or terbutaline 5–10 mg, but the delivered dose to the lung can be

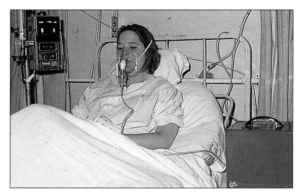

Fig 17.10. Acute asthmatic in hospital receiving oxygen, nebulised β-agonist and intravenous hydrocortisone and aminophylline. High dose inhaled β-agonists may usually be delivered safely from nebulisers driven by portable air compressors, but if the PaO_2 is low, the patient should also receive oxygen. Intravenous aminophylline may be associated with toxicity in severe asthma, if the patient has previously been on a methylxanthine and/or aminophylline is given by a fast intravenous injection. In this young asthmatic the intravenous therapy is delivered by a controlled intravenous infusion pump.

affected by the nebuliser/delivery system and gas flow rate (*see* Chapter 10). The response to a large dose of nebulised salbutamol is usually rapid, with marked improvement in PEF and the associated signs of severity of asthma, but this response should be maintained by further treatment. Family practitioners attending patients with acute severe asthma who are not able to deliver high-dose β-agonists via nebulisers may use a large volume spacer device and recommend the patient to actuate a standard dose pMDI every 30–60 seconds for up to 25 doses, as this is equivalent to the inhaled dose of drug recommended for the treatment of acute severe asthma delivered by a nebuliser.

Subcutaneous salbutamol or terbutaline may be effective if given before or during transfer to hospital. Intravenous β-agonists can be given by slow injection or, preferably, as a continuous intravenous infusion in hospital, but they are associated with an increased incidence of side effects and a greater chance of arterial hypoxaemia.

Anticholinergic agents

Ipratropium bromide has a role in the management of patients with severe asthma, despite its slower onset of action than inhaled β-agonists. Combination with β-agonists may produce a better bronchodilator response than either drug alone, and many accident and emergency departments tend to give the combination of anticholinergic and β-agonist as first-line treatment, or as the follow-up treatment after β-agonists. Ipratropium bromide is nebulised at a dose of 0.25–0.5 mg, but is not usually given as sole primary treatment because of its potential for bronchoconstriction.

Methylxanthines

Aminophylline has been given by slow intravenous injection in the treatment of severe acute asthma for many years. Inhaled high-dose β-agonist therapy has been shown to be as effective with fewer side effects so β-agonists are tending to replace methylxanthines as the initial treatment for severe asthma. Methylxanthines may increase side effects following high-dose β-agonist therapy. However, in the severely ill patient or the patient who is responding poorly to inhaled β-agonist therapy, aminophylline may be recommended as a slow intravenous injection over at least 20 minutes (5 mg/kg × body weight) followed by continuous infusion (0.5 mg/kg/hour) (**Fig. 17.9**). Nausea is common, with potentially fatal toxic effects if aminophylline serum levels exceed 30 μg/L. Serum theophylline levels should be estimated after the first 24 hours to prevent toxic

levels. Patients previously on oral methylxanthines should be given reduced loading doses and an early serum theophylline estimation. For a few patients intravenous aminophylline is associated with excellent therapeutic response, but in many guidelines it is now considered as a third-line bronchodilator.

Steroids

Steroids are recommended in the treatment of patients with acute asthma who do not respond rapidly and substantially to bronchodilator therapy. Intravenous hydrocortisone or methylprednisolone may be used, but in most cases extremely large doses are unnecessary. A dose of hydrocortisone (or methylprednisolone) which produces blood levels exceeding the levels achieved by stress has been suggested. Such levels are exceeded by hydrocortisone 3–4 mg/kg followed by the same dose 6-hourly (an empirical regimen of 200 mg followed by 200 mg 4–6 hourly is simpler and more frequently used). Methylprednisolone in a dose of 50–100 mg 12-hourly has also been recommended. Intravenous corticosteroids may be replaced by oral prednisolone in doses of 30–60 mg in most patients within 24–48 hours.

Patients with less severe acute asthma may be started on oral prednisolone (40–60 mg daily) with nebulised β-agonist. As the patient recovers, reduction in the dose of systemic/oral steroids should be associated with the early introduction of inhaled steroids, as long as they are not associated with cough or bronchoconstriction.

Assisted ventilation

Assisted ventilation is required in up to 2% of asthma admissions and may be a life-saving procedure. In adults a power cycled ventilator should be used with a cuffed endotracheal tube (**Fig. 17.11**). Indications for assisted ventilation (**Fig. 17.12**) tend to be imprecise. In some patients elective ventilation is carried out, in others it is forced upon the clinician. Systemic hypotension and physical exhaustion (a feature of prolonged acute severe asthma attacks) is a dangerous combination and if there is any doubt it is wiser to ventilate rather than wait for a respiratory or cardiorespiratory arrest. A $PaCO_2$ of 6.6 kPa and rising, a poorly maintained PaO_2 (falling) despite increases in the inspired oxygen concentration and respiratory acidosis suggest the need for ventilatory support. A potentially dangerous complication of intermittent positive pressure ventilation is tension pneumothorax.

The degree of barotrauma may, however, be over-estimated as the airway narrowing reduces the transfer of the high inflation pressure to the alveoli. Care should be taken to position the endotracheal tube correctly (**Figs 17.13, 17.14**) and allow an expiratory phase long enough to allow deflation of each tidal volume, otherwise air trapping will lead to systemic hypotension due to cardiac tamponade.

Additional measures

Antibiotic therapy is not routine in severe asthma but if a patient has purulent sputum during the onset of severe asthma then an antibiotic may be appropriate.

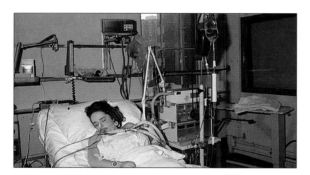

Fig. 17.11. Ventilation of a severely ill asthmatic. Asthma requiring intermittent positive ventilation is rare but may occur in all age groups. In this patient a falling PaO$_2$ in the presence of a rising PaCO$_2$ necessitated supportive ventilation to prevent respiratory arrest. Considerable difficulties can occur with supportive ventilation. Inspiratory time needs to be kept short compared with expiratory time to prevent gas trapping, while small inspiratory volumes help to prevent excessive airway pressures. Supportive ventilation corrects hypoxaemia and prevents hypercapnia from respiratory exhaustion whilst 'buying time' for bronchodilators and steroids to work. Over-zealous reduction in PaCO$_2$ is unnecessary and dangerous. Careful monitoring of arterial blood gases, ventilation volumes and pressures are used to assess recovery from asthma.

Indications for assisted ventilation

- PaCO$_2$ more than 50 mmHg (6.6 kPa) and rising
- PaO$_2$ less than 50 mmHg (6.6 kPa) and falling
- pH 7.3 or less and falling

Fig. 17.12. Indications for assisted ventilation.

Acute asthma may also be associated with yellow sputum due to the presence of eosinophils or casts (**Fig. 7.4**). Amoxycillin (or erythromycin in penicillin-allergic patients) is appropriate. Antibiotic therapy alone, without additional bronchodilator and oral steroids, should never be given. Although plugging of bronchi by tenacious mucus is a feature of severe acute asthma (**Fig. 2.5**) there is no evidence to suggest mucolytics are helpful. A high dose β-agonist, although primarily used to increase airway calibre, may be helpful in increasing the rate of clearance of bronchial mucus.

The mechanical removal of mucus plugs by bronchial lavage with saline, either via tracheal catheter or bronchoscopy, has been suggested in patients on intermittent positive pressure ventilation. However, serious bronchopulmonary infections have been reported and patients with acute severe asthma should not undergo bronchial lavage.

Physiotherapy may be counterproductive in the early phase of acute severe asthma, as persistent coughing tends to be associated with bronchoconstriction. During the recovery phase, as the airways dilate, most asthmatics have little difficulty in coughing up the sputum and bronchial casts voluntarily.

RECOVERY PHASE

Patients with acute severe asthma who do not require hospital admission are treated with oral steroids (around 30 mg prednisolone daily) for up to 2 weeks. Steroids can be tailed down progressively, but this is no longer considered essential if the course of steroids is for less than 3 weeks. It is less confusing for the patient if the steroid is stopped abruptly. An increase in inhaled steroids (or their introduction in patients not previously on inhaled steroids) should occur during the first week of the acute attack. High doses of β-agonist are reduced as the patient recovers, this recovery being monitored by diary card and peak-flow monitoring at home.

Patients admitted to hospital

There is a potential risk that, during recovery, patients will be given an over-rapid reduction in treatment. Transfer from high-dose β-agonists given via nebulisers to metered-dose aerosols may be associated with too rapid a reduction in dose (**Fig. 17.15**). During the recovery phase some asthmatics show an exaggerated morning dip with large swings in the diurnal variation of peak flow (**Fig. 17.16**). These can lead to cardiorespiratory arrest and death. This is particularly important in adult asthmatics where slow onset attacks may be associated with

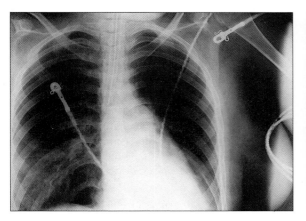

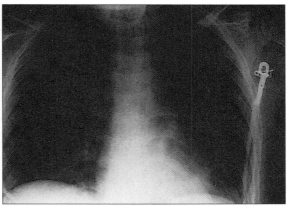

Figs 17.13, 17.14. Intubation of the right main bronchus. Patients arriving in the emergency room or on the ward with acute respiratory failure and cardiorespiratory arrest require rapid resuscitation. Intubation of the right main bronchus may occur (**17.13**) with consequent over-inflation of the right lung and progressive collapse of the left lower lobe with loss of lung volume. The cardiac silhouette is deviated to the left with deviation of the trachea to the left and loss of the left costophrenic angle. Extubation or resiting the endotracheal tube to the mid-trachea followed by gentle physiotherapy will lead to re-expansion of the left lung (**Fig. 17.14**).

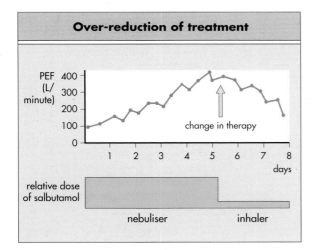

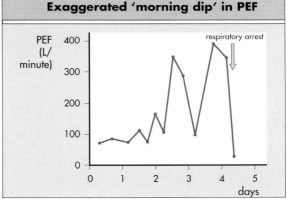

Fig. 17.16. Recovery pattern following an acute asthmatic attack in hospital. During the recovery phase from acute severe asthma some patients have an exaggerated 'morning dip' in the PEF. This may be associated with persistent hypoxaemia and the mechanism is believed to be that the large central airways are responding to therapy with bronchodilatation and reduced inflammatory activity more rapidly than the smaller more peripheral airways. Patients may still have poor gas exchange with a lower PaO_2 because of continued small airway bronchoconstriction and persistent inflammation with mucus plugging. Small changes in central airway bronchoconstriction could be associated with large falls in PEF and in the presence of maintained hypoxaemia are potentially fatal. Large swings in PEF are dangerous and associated with cardiorespiratory arrest and death.

Fig. 17.15. Over-reduction in treatment in an acute asthmatic who was rapidly changed from nebulised to pressurised aerosol bronchodilator. After 3–4 days in hospital the patient's peak flow and other symptoms all suggest a recovery from acute severe asthma. However, PEF fell progressively following the substitution of pMDI for nebulised bronchodilator. This worsening reflects the difference in dosage delivered by each system. Rapid reduction in bronchodilatation leads to a worsening in asthma and should be avoided. A progressive decrease in dose should be achieved by reducing the frequency of high-dose nebulised β-agonist, and the introduction of an inhaled β-agonist in higher dose and with higher lung delivery (e.g. by Turbuhaler) will result in a less abrupt reduction in therapy.

considerable airway inflammation and peripheral airway plugging. Too precipitate a discharge may occur, particularly in winter when there is pressure on hospital beds, and is frequently associated with increased readmission rates to hospital during the month after discharge. Safer discharge occurs (**Fig. 17.17**) when the diurnal variation between best and worst PEF is reduced to less than 20% and the patient's mean PEF is either 75% of their predicted or the best achieved recently.

Discharge

Before discharge the clinician should consider why the patient developed an acute attack of asthma. Pneumonia or other infections are easily identified precipitating factors. Environmental factors including weather may lead to an acute asthma attack. In June 1994 in the UK, a combination of a week of hot weather and a sudden increase in humidity followed by thunderstorms (**Fig. 6.8**), was followed by an epidemic of acute asthma admission. High levels of vehicle emissions, both nitrous oxide and particulate emissions, were also recorded. The

mechanism for this epidemic has not been fully explained but sensitisation of airways by such vehicle emissions and subsequent increased susceptibility to allergens is likely. The high humidity would lead to disintegration of grass and fungal spore pollens giving fragments of a size which could be inhaled rather than deposited in the upper airways. The fact that weather conditions can lead to an increase in the number of admissions for acute severe asthma has been also documented in the USA and Spain.

Changes within the local environment, e.g. new pet, new home, new job, or additional stress should be looked for (*see* Chapter 6). Often, however, acute attacks are associated with a reduction in compliance with prescribed medication or a failure to renew supplies of prescribed medication. Patients should be discharged with clearly written instructions regarding medication and an overall self-management plan (*see* Chapter 12). Inhaler technique should be checked to ensure effective use of the device. Follow-up may be at hospital or primary care level, but it is important that there is continuity of care.

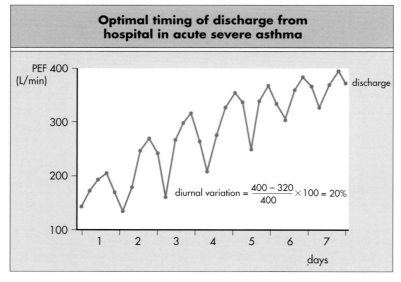

Fig. 17.17. When to discharge to prevent a significant chance of re-admission. After admission for an acute severe asthma attack the pattern of recovery in PEF is associated with a progressive increase in midday to late afternoon PEF, but a maintained morning dip (see **Fig. 17.16**). Over the first 3–4 days following admission the maximum daily PEF may rise to near the patient's predicted or best, but premature discharge at this stage is associated with a greater chance of re-admission with asthma in the succeeding month. Ideally patients should not be discharged until the diurnal variation is less than 20%, as is shown here, and the best peak flow is within 75% of the predicted PEF or the best PEF the patient has recorded recently.

18 SPECIAL SITUATIONS

EXERCISE-INDUCED ASTHMA

The development of an acute asthma attack following a short period of exercise is a common problem in many patients with asthma. The degree of severity varies with the type of exercise, and free running often leads to more severe exacerbations than cycling or swimming. The temperature and humidity of the inspired air can also affect the severity of the attack. Simple exercise testing may be used in children and young adults for diagnosis of asthma (**Figs 14.13, 14.14, 18.1**). Typically after 6 minutes running there will be a fall in PEF (**Fig. 18.2**). The mechanism for exercise-induced asthma has been disputed (**Fig. 18.3**).

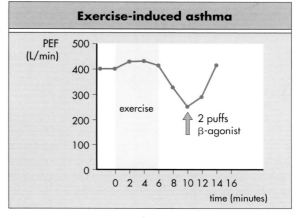

Fig. 18.2. Treatment of isolated shortness of breath after exercise in young adults. Confirmation of exercise-induced asthma by carrying out a 6-minute vigorous exercise test on a treadmill or with free running is the most potent stimulus. Measuring PEF during, and for 15 minutes after the exercise, is useful. Exercise-induced asthma may be reduced or prevented by premedication 15 minutes before exercise with β-agonists or sodium cromoglycate or reversed by an inhaled post-exercise β-agonist. If exercise-induced asthma persists then an increase in pre-exercise β-agonist may be tried.

Fig. 18.1. Measuring the PEF response to exercise testing. Exercise should be vigorous, and should last for about 6 minutes. Responses can be enhanced by exercising in cold, dry air.

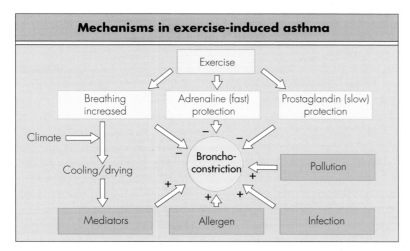

Fig. 18.3. Some suggested pathways involved in exercise-induced asthma. Exercise leads to increased ventilation, producing cooling and drying of the airways. This trigger liberates bronchoconstrictor mediators, the degree of bronchoconstriction induced varying with the degree of bronchial hyperresponsiveness and level of allergen stimulation. During exercise, bronchoconstriction is opposed by adrenaline released by exercise, so most patients only develop bronchoconstriction after exercise has finished. Prostaglandins may also be released giving further protection from bronchoconstriction.

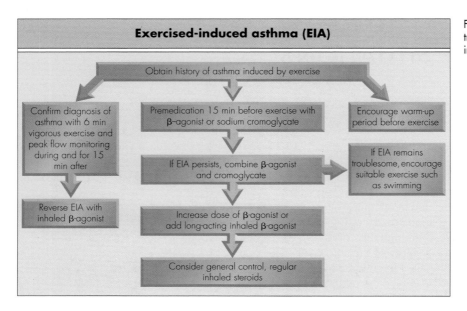

Fig. 18.4. Confirmation and treatment of exercise-induced asthma.

Increased ventilation leads to airway cooling and drying of the airway which triggers the liberation of bronchoconstrictor mediators. The degree of bronchoconstriction produced depends on the responsiveness of the airway and other factors, including the level of allergen stimulation while exercise is undertaken, and protection by naturally released adrenaline. In many asthmatics a second exercise challenge within 1 hour will produce a much smaller effect on the airways – so-called refractoriness.

Exercise-induced asthma may be blocked in the acute challenge by prior use of sodium cromoglycate, which has no bronchodilator effect, or with some pre-exercise bronchodilatation by inhaled β-agonist. The effects of theophylline and ipratropium bromide are less predictable. Inhaled steroids are not protective in an acute challenge, but if taken as long-term prophylactic treatment appear to reduce exercise-induced asthma.

Treatment of exercise-induced asthma is usually part of the overall treatment of asthma but in a few young adults it is the only significant symptom and the long-term use of inhaled anti-inflammatory drugs is likely to be associated with poor compliance. Confirmation of exercise-induced asthma is usually worthwhile and treatment consists of premedication with β-agonist or sodium cromoglycate 15 minutes before exercise. If problems remain the dose of β-agonist can be increased, a long-acting inhaled β-agonist can be added, or regular inhaled steroids given (**Fig. 18.4**). Changing to a less provocative exercise, such as swimming, is better than the patient doing no exercise because of asthma.

COMPETITIVE SPORT AND ASTHMA

Treating asthma and exercise-induced asthma in patients may allow the individual to be competitive at many sports but care should be taken not to use banned substances. In most countries there is a National Sports Council from which information about permitted and banned medication can be obtained. In the UK and most of Europe, inhaled steroids are allowed for both asthma and rhinitis. Most inhaled β-agonists, sodium cromoglycate and theophylline may also be taken. Oral β-stimulants are usually banned, especially clenbuterol which has an anabolic steroid like action on muscle. Olympic regulations are more stringent and may prevent an asthmatic competing at this level of competition.

NOCTURNAL ASTHMA

Wakening during the night with an acute attack of asthma is indicative of poor control, but many asthmatics believe it is a normal part of their life. Nocturnal wakening, although almost diagnostic of asthma in young adults, may have to be differentiated from acute pulmonary oedema ('cardiac asthma') where wheezing may be a prominent feature (**Fig. 18.5**) in the older patient. Clinical features of pulmonary oedema are the production of pink frothy sputum, with late inspiratory crackles heard on auscultation and radiological features of pulmonary oedema (**Fig. 8.13**). The frequency of nocturnal wakening is a good indicator of poor overall

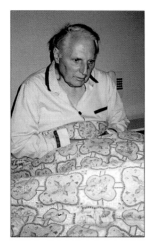

Fig. 18.5. Patient wakening with acute breathlessness at night. Waking acutely short of breath with severe wheeze is now accepted as a major indication of poor control in asthma. In young adults the diagnosis is simple, but in older patients nocturnal asthma may be confused with acute pulmonary oedema secondary to ischaemic or other heart disease. The prominence of the wheeze usually suggests asthma, while coughing productive of pink frothy sputum suggests pulmonary oedema.

Management of nocturnal asthma

- Monitor degree of problem with PEF measurements
- Check exposure to precipitating factors such as dust mite, pets, feather pillows/duvets
- Improve general control with regular prophylactic therapy: inhaled steroid, sodium cromoglycate or nedocromil
- Add long-acting β-agonist or ipratropium bromide by inhalation
- Add oral slow-release bronchodilator at bedtime (β-agonist or theophylline, measuring blood levels)
- Increase dose of inhaled steroid

Fig. 18.6. Management of nocturnal asthma.

control of asthma in most patients and adequate daytime control with prophylactic medication is usually all that is required to control nocturnal symptoms.

The mechanisms of nocturnal asthma have been extensively investigated and it is now considered to be associated with an exaggeration of the normal diurnal variation in airway reactivity, with changes in adrenaline, noradrenaline, histamine and endogenous steroid production as well as parasympathetic vagal stimulation. There is no simple relationship between these factors as changes in PEF occur rapidly in shift workers while changes related to the hypothalamic-pituitary-adrenal axis are slower to occur. Exposure to house dust mite or other allergens and the short length of action of many therapies have also been suggested as contributory factors.

Although in the majority of patients good daytime control of asthma using inhaled therapy will prevent nocturnal wakening, this remains a problem in a few patients.

Long-acting β₂-agonist in nocturnal asthma

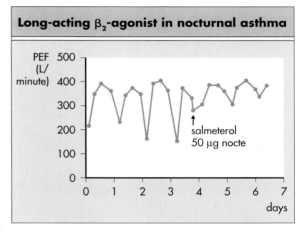

Fig. 18.7. Effect of introduction of a bedtime inhalation of salmeterol on PEF in a patient on regular inhaled steroids with no daytime symptoms of asthma. The frequency of nocturnal wakening also fell.

Treatment

Identifying the severity as well as the frequency of the nocturnal asthma is useful and at-home peak flow measurements should be considered. High levels of allergen exposure, particularly to the house dust mite, pets and feather pillows/duvets should be avoided. Regular inhaled prophylactic therapy and compliance should be reviewed (**Fig. 18.6**). Slow-release oral bronchodilators, either β-agonists or theophylline, or long-acting bambuterol may be considered and the long-acting inhaled β-agonists such as salmeterol and formoterol are particularly helpful (**Fig. 18.7**). Anticholinergic therapy may

also be considered and may be theoretically advantageous in the older patient.

INTERMITTENT SEVERE ASTHMA ('BRITTLE ASTHMA')

Intermittent severe asthma ('brittle asthma') is fortunately rare but tends to occur in children or young adults. It is characterised by the patient developing short catastrophic acute attacks of asthma with a fall in PEF in a matter of minutes from within the patient's normal range to being very low or unrecordable (**Fig. 18.8**). Patients frequently have a well-maintained peak flow between

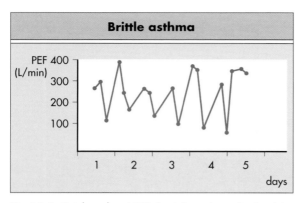

Fig. 18.8. 'Brittle asthma' PEF. Peak flow chart of a 'brittle' asthmatic who has wide variations in PEF, with her PEF falling precipitously in a matter of a few minutes leading to a catastrophic life-threatening attack of asthma. This patient had little perception of the severity of her attacks.

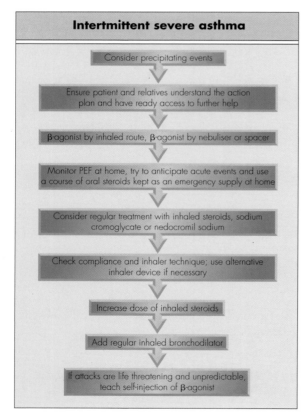

Fig. 18.9. Intermittent severe asthma ('brittle asthma'). Treatment of 'brittle asthma' may be difficult, particularly because of its catastrophic acute nature. However, recognising precipitating actions and trying to anticipate acute events are important. Frequent use of a pMDI may be effective but in some patients the attacks are life threatening and self-injection of β-agonists or adrenaline should be taught.

attacks. About 20% of asthma deaths occur in such patients. Treatment should start with careful consideration of any precipitating events so these can be avoided (**Fig. 18.9**). Upper respiratory tract viral infections can lead to unstable asthma, which may be recognised from PEF recordings allowing the patient to take appropriate action. Patients and relatives should be advised on a clear plan of action in an attack. At its simplest this is the repeated use of a pMDI of β-agonist, with or without a large volume spacer, while in the most severe acute attacks patients are advised on self-injection of β-agonists or adrenaline. Further acute attacks may occur so it is important that the patient starts a course of oral steroids (prednisolone 30–40 mg each morning for 1 week to 10 days) and continues higher doses of β-agonist, particularly during the first 24 hours following the acute attack.

CHRONIC SINUSITIS

Allergic rhinitis is commonly associated with asthma (**Fig. 18.10**) and in a few patients there may also be persistent sinus infection. Such patients with a post-nasal drip or persistently infected nasal passages may have their asthma dramatically improved by sinus drainage and clearing of any infected material. Antibiotics, antihistamines, nasal decongestants, topical anti-inflammatories and, in a minority, surgical drainage should be considered when chronic sinusitis is diagnosed.

ASTHMA AND PREGNANCY

Asthma complicates at least 1% of all pregnancies but usually has no serious implications to either the mother or fetus. Frequently, unless otherwise warned, a woman with asthma who wishes to become pregnant reduces or stops regular inhaled prophylactic medication on the basis that all drugs may damage the fetus. This will increase the risk of an acute attack of asthma and the need for systemic steroids. Potentially child-bearing asthmatics should be made aware of the comparative safety of β-agonists and inhaled steroids to the developing fetus (**Fig. 18.11**). Most studies suggest that hypoxia from an asthma attack is more likely to cause damage to the fetus than prophylactic therapy. Once conception has occurred the mother's asthma may stay the same, get worse, or get better, and the change in symptoms and PEF may vary through each of the trimesters. Most guidelines advise that specialist supervision of pregnant women with asthma is required, but it is important that the obstetrician, family practitioner and respiratory specialist liaise and co-ordinate the patient's care. Regular monitoring of peak flow with a self-management plan, and increasing and decreasing prophylactic medication following the changes in symptoms and PEF should be advised. Acute attacks of asthma should be treated conventionally ensuring high oxygen saturations and using prednisolone rather than hydrocortisone when possible. Prednisolone/methylprednisolone do not cross the placental barrier to any large degree, in contrast to hydrocortisone and dexamethasone, so if systemic steroids are required just before delivery it is unlikely that there will be suppression of the HPA axis of the fetus. Acute asthma during labour is uncommon but usually responds to high-dose β-agonists with systemic steroids. Inhaled medications usually do not affect breast milk (**Fig. 18.12**), but oral theophylline may be associated with neonatal hyperactivity.

Careful supervision, encouraging good compliance with medication during pregnancy and treating attacks early in a conventional way is likely to be associated with a successful outcome for both mother and child.

ASPIRIN-INDUCED ASTHMA

Aspirin-induced asthma has been recognised for nearly 100 years and more recently asthma has been noted to occur also with many non-steroidal anti-inflammatory agents, all of which act as cyclo-oxygenase inhibitors.

Bronchoconstriction develops within minutes to several hours of ingestion of aspirin or NSAID and may be associated with rhinorrhoea, flushing or loss of consciousness; it may be fatal.

Patients usually present in the second or third decade with intermittent watery rhinorrhoea which becomes more persistent with the development of nasal polyps (**Fig. 5.7**) and sinusitis. Asthmatic symptoms are increasingly obviously associated temporally with the ingestion of aspirin – an association that must be sought when taking the history. Aspirin challenge may be indicated in adult asthmatics who require NSAIDs for another medical problem and is safe as long as the oral challenge follows the recommended standardised protocol in hospital. The mechanism of aspirin-induced asthma is not fully understood but it has been found not to be related to inhibition of prostaglandin synthetase changing the products of metabolism of arachidonic acid as previously thought. Patients with a clear history of aspirin or NSAID bronchoconstriction should be warned to avoid aspirin and given a list of similar potentially asthma-provoking agents. Occasionally, salicylates in foods may cause symptoms. Paracetamol is an appropriate substitute simple analgesic although rare asthma-like reactions have also been reported to this drug. Patients who require aspirin and NSAID for other medical illness can be desensitised to aspirin under specialised supervision by the administration of repeated small oral doses of aspirin. Acute and chronic asthma in patients with aspirin sensitivity should be treated in the same way as other forms of asthma.

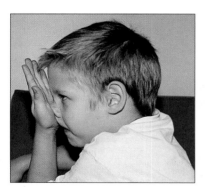

Fig. 18.10. Allergic rhinitis is commonly associated with asthma, especially in childhood. Occasionally, surgical treatment for associated chronic sinusitis may lead to a considerable improvement in the patient's asthma.

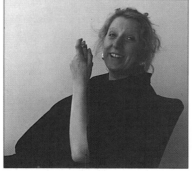

Fig. 18.11. Asthma and pregnancy. Hypoxia from an acute attack is more likely to cause fetal damage than prophylactic inhaled therapy. Inhaled therapy should usually be continued through conception and pregnancy.

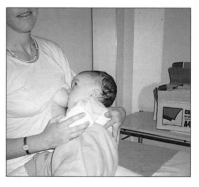

Fig. 18.12. Inhaled therapy in asthma is not usually a contraindication to breast feeding. Inhaled medications do not usually reach breast milk in significant concentrations. Maternal oral theophylline therapy may, however, lead to hyperactivity in a breastfed infant.

INDEX